EBOLA

Profile of a Killer Virus

DOROTHY H. CRAWFORD

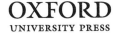

OXFORD

UNIVERSITY PRESS

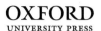

UNIVERSITY PRESS

Great Clarendon Street, Oxford, OX2 6DP,
United Kingdom

Oxford University Press is a department of the University of Oxford.
It furthers the University's objective of excellence in research, scholarship,
and education by publishing worldwide. Oxford is a registered trade mark of
Oxford University Press in the UK and in certain other countries

© Dorothy H. Crawford 2016

The moral rights of the author have been asserted

First Edition published in 2016
Impression: 1

Published in the United States of America by Oxford University Press
198 Madison Avenue, New York, NY 10016, United States of America

British Library Cataloguing in Publication Data
Data available

Library of Congress Control Number: 2016943467

ISBN 978–0–19–875999–7

Printed in Great Britain by
Clays Ltd, St Ives plc

This book is dedicated to Dr Jean Alero Thomas (1945–2015)

ACKNOWLEDGEMENTS

I would like to thank all those experts who helped and advised on the writing of this book: Tim Brooks, Public Health England, Jeremy Farrar, Wellcome Trust, Ian Goodfellow, University of Cambridge, Brian Greenwood, London School of Hygiene and Tropical Medicine, David Heymann, Public Health England and Centre on Global Health Security, Paul Johnson, Public Health England, Peter Piot, London School of Hygiene and Tropical Medicine, and Katrina Roper, World Health Organization.

I am also indebted to the following for reading and commenting on the manuscript: William Alexander, Martin Allday, Jeanne Bell, Richard Boyd, Jude Fantes, Tanzina Haque, Ingolfur Johannessen, Barbara Judge, Jim Piper, Iain Ritchie, Paul Saba, Bobby Stansfield, Tara Womersley, and to Latha Menon at Oxford University Press for her constant support.

I am particularly grateful to Frances Fowler, who facilitated my meetings with Ebola experts, and Tim Brooks, who allowed me to shadow him for a short time while he went about his busy schedule in Sierra Leone in April 2015.

CONTENTS

LIST OF FIGURES

ABBREVIATIONS

AD3	Chimpanzee adenovirus 3
AIDS	Acquired immune deficiency syndrome
CDC	Centres for Disease Control
DNA	Deoxyribonucleic acid
DRC	Democratic Republic of Congo
EM	Electron microscope
Flu	Influenza
GAVI	Global Alliance Vaccine Initiative
GDP	Gross domestic product
HIV	Human immunodeficiency virus
MRI	Magnetic resonance imaging
MSF	Médècins Sans Frontières (Doctors without Borders)
MVA	Modified vaccinia Ankara virus
NGO	Non-governmental organization
PCR	Polymerase chain reaction
PHE	Public Health England
PLZ	Lever Plantations in Zaire
RNA	Ribonucleic acid
SARS	Severe acute respiratory syndrome
TB	Tuberculosis
UNICEF	United Nations International Children's Emergency Fund
VSV	Vesicular stomatitis virus
WHO	World Health Organization

INTRODUCTION

When I arrived in Freetown, Sierra Leone, in April 2015 the atmosphere was electric. There was clear optimism in the air; the Ebola epidemic that had been raging for more than a year was coming under control, markets were functioning again, and schools had reopened. But no one could miss the fact that the country was in the grip of a deadly epidemic. At the airport we were politely told to wash our hands in chlorine solution even before entering the building. Once inside we completed long health questionnaires and were submitted to health checks. Gowned and masked figures wearing plastic gloves and aprons took our temperatures using a Thermoflash—a handgun-shaped, electronic, infrared, contactless thermometer—alarmingly aimed straight at the forehead.

This ritual of hand washing and temperature taking was repeated numerous times during my stay. Vats of chlorine solution sat outside every building, be it a hospital, office block, supermarket, or hotel. No one was allowed to enter without washing their hands and having their temperature taken. The same ritual occurred at

1

frequent intervals along the highways; my temperature remained stubbornly at 36.2°C throughout.

All over the country Ebola had a palpable presence. Everyone was committed to abolishing the deadly virus. Freetown was ringed by police check points to ensure no Ebola victim could evade quarantine. Streets were lined with Ebola posters with catchy reminders:

> ABC—AVOID BODY CONTACT
> NHS—NO HAND SHAKES
> EBOLA STOPS WITH ME!

While in Sierra Leone I accompanied Dr Tim Brooks from Public Health England as he visited treatment centres and supervised the Ebola testing laboratories he had set up for the UK Government. I met UK and Sierra Leonean government officials, frontline health care workers, laboratory technicians, and epidemiologists, all brave people dedicated to one cause—ridding the country of Ebola. This firsthand experience of the Ebola response proved invaluable when writing this book.

In Freetown I stayed at the Radisson Hotel and so, it seemed, did everyone else. The hotel was full of Response Teams from World Health Organization, UNICEF, the US Centres for Disease Control, Médècins Sans Frontières, Oxfam, and Save the Children as well as experts and non-governmental organization (NGO) staff from China, Canada, South Africa, and many other countries, all working single-mindedly in pursuit of the same goal—complete Ebola eradication. Yet, at least to the uninitiated, each team seemed to be working individually with no one in overall control and no all-inclusive, logically organized response plan. I soon gave up trying to make sense of it; the bottom line was that at last the response was working.

* * *

The first recorded Ebola outbreak occurred in a remote village in the Democratic Republic of Congo (DRC) in 1976. Appearing as if from nowhere, the previously unknown disease killed 280 of the 318 villagers it infected before disappearing again just as mysteriously. But the curiously long, thread-like Ebola disease virus that caused this devastating outbreak has reappeared many times over the years to decimate other communities, mostly in remote corners of Africa, and then vanished again just as promptly. At least twenty-four African communities have suffered Ebola outbreaks, all following a similar pattern—the sudden appearance of a rapidly spreading plague that kills most of its victims before departing again leaving the stricken survivors to rebuild their lives.

Like many tropical diseases, Ebola has been neglected by medical researchers, perhaps because it had always proved either self-limiting or fairly easy to eradicate using public health measures alone. In 2011, this comforting thought prompted me to write: 'Counter-intuitively, control of Ebola outbreaks is quite straightforward once the disease is recognised. Since the infection is so debilitating, few infected victims move far from the outbreak site and once the person-to-person chain of infection is broken by strict barrier nursing and isolation of cases and contacts, it can be rapidly controlled.'[1]

All this changed in West Africa in 2014. Ebola displayed a frightening new pattern of infection, shifting from a rural to an urban plague. In the cities of Guinea, Sierra Leone, and Liberia the virus spread easily and quickly, infecting and killing more people in this one epidemic than it had ever killed before, and proving extremely difficult to eradicate.

This book covers the whole history of Ebola from the initial outbreak in 1976 to the unique and devastating epidemic of 2014–16. The first three chapters introduce Ebola virus and the disease it causes, and describe the Ebola outbreaks and their control prior to 2014. But most of the book (Chapters 4–9) focuses on the Ebola epidemic centred in the West African countries of Liberia, Sierra Leone, and Guinea in 2014–16. Using data from scientific studies interspersed with personal accounts from researchers, virus experts, public health officials, and health care workers, we track the deadly disease as it spreads from the initial outbreak site in rural Guinea and evolves into the largest ever Ebola epidemic. For the first time the virus spread to several countries, its impact felt far beyond the African continent. We follow the national and international attempts to control the epidemic and pinpoint exactly where and when it all began. We discuss the questions of where the virus came from, why it spread so widely, the identity of the animal that hosts the virus between human outbreaks, and why Ebola moved from its traditional territory in Central Africa to strike in West Africa.

In Chapter 8 we look at the Ebola drug and vaccine trials that eventually got underway in West Africa, and debate the sensitive ethical issues surrounding the design of clinical trials of experimental products during such a lethal epidemic. The final chapter discusses the legacy of devastation left by Ebola in Guinea, Sierra Leone, and Liberia, which goes far beyond the confines of Ebola itself. It is imperative that the shattered health services in the region are urgently rebuilt. Only then will basic health care facilities for maternal and child health and control of malaria, HIV, and many other fatal diseases be restored. The 2014–16 Ebola epidemic highlighted several defects in global health security. It is clear that until *every* country has a functional early warning system to detect outbreaks of lethal diseases such as Ebola the whole world is vulnerable. We have to be prepared for all eventualities if we are to prevent another humanitarian crisis.

1

When Disaster Strikes

The First Ebola Outbreak

Ebola—the very name evokes fear and panic. And no wonder, because Ebola is the virus of horror movies and nightmares. It appears as if from nowhere, striking suddenly and unpredictably, and produces agonizing symptoms. And with no specific treatment available, it kills over half its victims. Until 2014 most people in the world had never heard of Ebola, but the epidemic in West Africa changed all that by posing a global threat.

The first Ebola outbreak ever recorded occurred four decades ago in a remote village in Zaire (Zaire is now called the Democratic Republic of Congo (DRC)). Although the virus may have struck isolated communities in Central Africa before this, all previous outbreaks went unnoticed by the outside world. Perhaps even locally the deadly effects of Ebola were unrecognizable against a background of killer microbes that target poor and isolated communities in Sub Saharan Africa. Diseases like malaria, gastroenteritis, acute respiratory infection, measles, smallpox, and Acquired Immunodeficiency Syndrome (AIDS) all share the non-specific symptoms of early Ebola, and generally these infections are, or, in the case of smallpox, have been, far more common. But when Ebola strikes no one is safe. Left to its own devices the virus rips through a community killing the majority of its victims. And then it disappears—only to reappear at another time in another place.

DRC is one of the largest countries in Africa—the size of Western Europe. Its capital, Kinshasa, is strategically placed on the Congo River basin in the southwest corner of the country. In the 1970s the country was sparsely populated, with around 20 million inhabitants (DRC now has a population of ~80 million). The village of Yambuku lies in the northern Bumba Zone of the Equateur Region of DRC (Figure 1), a region of dense, tropical rain forest. Yambuku is 1089km (677 miles) from Kinshasa, and even today the village is remote and neglected. Villagers belong to the Budza tribe and speak the local Budza language and/or the more widespread Lingala.

Yambuku is famous for just one thing—Ebola. In 1976 the virus struck, infecting 318 villagers and killing 280 of them. Through a combination of historical links and lucky coincidences, this outbreak attracted international attention. A full investigation followed, which identified a new disease, Ebola haemorrhagic fever (now renamed Ebola virus disease) and its cause—Ebola disease virus.

* * *

Yambuku 1976—the village is unique among the cluster of villages in the area for having a small Catholic mission set up by Belgian missionaries in 1935—one of seven in the Bumba Zone. The mission includes a church, a hospital, and a school with a community of seven nuns, Sisters of the Sacred Heart of Our Lady of s'Gravenwezel (a small town in Belgium), three priests, and around sixty resident families. The nuns run a 120-bed hospital where they act

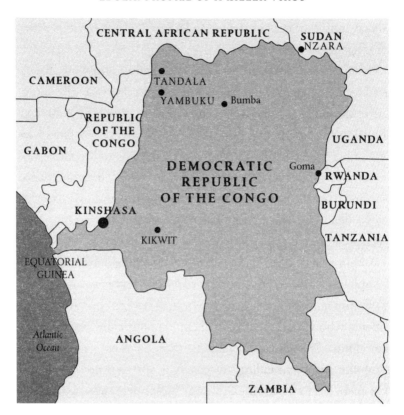

Figure 1 Map of Democratic Republic of Congo showing location of early Ebola outbreaks.

as nurses and midwives, aided by a staff of fourteen, including a medical assistant. Since these provide the only medical facilities for miles around, and the hospital is generally well stocked with medicines, villagers from the surrounding area frequently visit the clinic at Yambuku Mission Hospital. In all it serves around 60,000 people and treats as many as 12,000 a month. But with no doctors or trained laboratory workers, the clinic staff have no means of making firm diagnoses. So treatment is handed out on an empirical basis. All seems very orderly in this quiet, isolated village, but then disaster strikes and Yambuku is never quite the same again.

On August 26, 1976, the 44-year-old Yambuku mission school head teacher, Mabalo Lokela, develops a fever. He visits the clinic where the nuns assume he has malaria and give him a shot of chloroquine. Following this his fever resolves, but then on September 1 he falls ill again. When he returns to the clinic on September 5, he is admitted to the hospital with diarrhoea and bleeding from the nose. Here his symptoms worsen, he develops a severe headache and abdominal pains, copious vomiting, and widespread bleeding. He dies in the hospital on September 8.

Within a week of Lokela's death nine more Yambuku villagers die, apparently from the same disease. First, members of the teacher's family fall ill, then the nuns who had treated him and other patients who visited the mission hospital on the day he attended the clinic. The dreadful disease then sweeps on through Yambuku and surrounding villages, typically causing high fever, skin rash, severe headache and abdominal pain, uncontrollable diarrhoea and vomiting, and both internal and external bleeding— leading to an agonizing death in almost every case.

When two nuns at the mission die of the disease the others begin to panic. They send out a plea for help and a doctor from the District capital, Bumba, visits on September 16 followed, on September 21, by infectious disease experts from Kinshasa. They suspect an outbreak of typhoid fever and so when two more nuns, Sisters Myriam and Edmunda, fall ill they are airlifted to the capital for treatment. On September 25 they are admitted to the private Clinique Ngaliema in Kinshasa under the care of Dr Jacques Courteille, the Belgian Director of Internal Medicine. The two nuns rapidly succumb to the mystery illness.

Courteille is baffled by the nuns' symptoms but thinks that they must have a severe form of yellow fever. This disease, caused by yellow fever virus, is endemic in tropical and subtropical Africa where it is spread by *Aedes aegypti* mosquitoes. It usually causes an illness similar to a bad bout of 'flu with fever, general malaise, loss of appetite, headache, and muscle pains, lasting around five days. But in approximately 10% of cases this progresses to haemorrhagic fever with internal bleeding that may cause tissue injury. Liver damage produces the jaundice (yellowing of the skin) that gives the disease its name. Although the nuns have been vaccinated against yellow fever virus, Courteille still thinks that this is the most likely diagnosis. Fortunately though, he decides to send a blood sample from one of the nuns to the Prince Leopold Institute of Tropical Medicine in Antwerp, Belgium, for confirmatory testing.

Back in Yambuku, the plague continues its unrelenting course. At first it is confined to those who visit the clinic, including several pregnant women as well as mothers and their newborn infants. Then it spreads to their families, friends, and relations. Many flee the area in the hope of escaping almost certain death. And so the disease reaches outlying villages; fifty-five of the 250 within a 120km (~75-mile) radius of Yambuku eventually report cases of *Yambuku fever*, as the disease is now known locally.[1] In a few villages the elders remember procedures enforced during the intensive smallpox eradication campaign of the 1960s and early 1970s and erect a crude *cordon sanitaire*, or barrier, around their villages to prevent people entering or leaving. Despite this, several people escape, fleeing as far as Bumba, some 120km away, reaching there in early October.

The nuns at the mission have no idea what has caused this plague and are at a loss to know what to do about it. In seeking a reason for it they wonder if its appearance is linked to recent events. In particular, the head teacher had returned from a trip in the forest just a few days before the onset of his illness. As he brought some bush meat back with him, they think that this might have been contaminated with a toxin that kick-started the Yambuku fever outbreak. On the other hand, noting the large number of newborns dying of the disease, they suggest that this might relate to a recent rise in stillbirths among their herd of pigs. But none of this musing tells them what to do, and as the disease spreads in an ever widening circle, the nuns, distraught with grief and fear, are at their wits' end to know how to stop it.

By the end of September most of the villagers are either dead or have fled the area. At the mission eleven of the seventeen staff and thirty-nine members of the mission families have died and the rest have absconded. Only one elderly priest, Father Léon, the Mother Superior, Sister Marcella, and two nuns, Sisters Genoveva and Mariette, are left alive, and they expect to follow their sisters and brothers to their death beds imminently. Like the village elders, they know that in an epidemic a *cordon sanitaire* should be erected to prevent the disease spreading. And so on October 3, the nuns close the hospital, then string a cord around the premises, nail a notice to a tree saying in Lingala: 'Anyone who passes this fence will die', and retreat to their guesthouse to prepare themselves for death.[2]

Meanwhile, in Bumba, the coffee and rice harvests should be in full swing with the produce being shipped down the Congo River to Kinshasa for export. But when rumours of a plague of Yambuku fever reach the town, and then plague-sufferers themselves start to arrive, the whole zone is quarantined by the Minister of Health and placed under martial law. The port is silent and the small airstrip which, along with the river, is their life line to the outside world, is out of action. Spooked pilots have returned to Kinshasa reporting dead bodies lying everywhere in Bumba, and thereafter they refuse to fly there. Fear, panic, and then hunger take hold and angry crowds have to be controlled by military police.

Similarly, at the Lever Plantations in Zaire (PLZ) headquarters in Ebonda 10km from Bumba, staff are panicking. Unilever own most of the thriving coffee, cocoa, palm oil, rubber, and rice plantations in the area, and now the staff are desperate for help and advice. Not only are they banned from transporting their harvested produce, but they are also running out of essential supplies of food and medicines. Several members of their employees' families are either dead or dying from Yambuku fever and they have no idea how to treat them or to handle the bodies for burial.

* * *

By sending blood samples from the sick nun to the Prince Leopold Institute of Tropical Medicine in Belgium, Courteille inadvertently alerted the world to the Yambuku fever outbreak. For him the Institute was a natural choice since DRC had been a Belgian colony—the Belgian Congo—until it gained independence in 1960. (After independence the Belgian Congo was renamed Zaire. It became DRC in 1997.) The Institute was founded in 1906 specifically to train doctors for work in the colonies and to carry out research into the tropical diseases that they battled against. Historic links remained and so Courteille sent the samples to Professor Stefaan Pattyn, a microbiologist at the Institute. By mid-October a completely new virus had been discovered in the nun's blood sample in Belgium; the story of the isolation and characterization of this virus is detailed in Chapter 2. The idea of a new killer virus on the loose was enough to stimulate the Zairian Government to hastily convene an International Commission to investigate the outbreak, and on October 18, Commission members touched down in Kinshasa ready to start work.

Amongst the Commission members was Peter Piot (now Director of the London School of Hygiene and Tropical Medicine), then a 27-year-old trainee virologist working with Pattyn at the Prince Leopold Institute of Tropical Medicine. He was one of the team in Pattyn's laboratory that isolated the new virus and he was determined to witness the situation on the ground in Zaire. He and Pattyn flew to Kinshasa where they met up with experts from the World Health Organization (WHO), the US Centers for Disease Control (CDC), France, and South Africa, as well as the Zairian Minister of Health and a Professor of Microbiology from Kinshasa, Jean-Jaques Muyembe, the only one of the group who had already visited Yambuku.

The Commission's priority was to prevent an epidemic of Yambuku fever in Kinshasa. In this overcrowded and chaotic city medical and administrative infrastructure was almost non-existent, corruption was a way of life, and most of the three million inhabitants believed that the rule of law was there to be flouted. A rogue virus on the loose was everyone's worst nightmare. And with the recent deaths of Sisters Myriam and Edmunda in the city, the Commissioners knew that this was a definite possibility. But then they received even more alarming news; on October 12, a nurse who had looked after the Yambuku nuns at the Clinique, called Mayinga N'Seka, developed high fever and headache. She was admitted to the ward where her symptoms progressed to the typical bleeding, diarrhoea, and vomiting of

Yambuku fever. At the very moment that the Commission met for the first time she was fighting for her life nearby. Now they deemed further spread of the lethal virus in the city to be highly likely.

The mood at the Clinique was one of alarm bordering on panic. Without any knowledge of how this lethal virus spread to others, the staff observed strict safety precautions. Dressed in spacesuit-like protective clothing, they burned the contaminated mattresses used by the deceased nuns, fumigated their rooms, and wrapped their bodies in sheets soaked in strong disinfectant. They then sealed them in double body bags before placing them in coffins. Mayinga's contacts were urgently traced and quarantined. In the end fourteen medical staff from the affected ward along with thirty-seven contacts and family members were detained and isolated until the danger was over. As it happened Mayinga had recently paid a visit to the Ministry of Foreign Affairs regarding a student visa application for study abroad, and so ministry staff were among those quarantined. As one member of the Commission commented, this was 'potentially the most deadly epidemic of the century'.[3]

The Commission urgently disseminated advice for diagnosing and dealing with suspected cases of Yambuku fever to all medical personnel in Zaire as well as information on protective clothing for health care workers and case isolation procedures. At the same time a National Surveillance Team was set up in Kinshasa for immediate investigation of suspected cases. And, as an indication as to how seriously the Commission took the threat, a portable, negative-pressure bed isolator was flown in from Canada and set up in Clinique Ngaliema to accommodate any proven Yambuku fever cases.

Although, sadly, nurse Mayinga died, all this frenetic activity paid off. Despite many alerts, all the possible cases reported turned out to be false alarms, and there were no more Yambuku fever cases in Kinshasa. This was fortunate indeed, since in this urban setting Ebola virus spread would have been virtually impossible to control.

*   *   *

Despite his young age and inexperience, Piot was chosen to be one of a small Commission subgroup sent to Yambuku ahead of the full international team to make a preliminary report. On October 19, the subgroup were flown to Bumba (by very reluctant pilots!) and driven from there through the rain forest to Yambuku. They arrived on the scene to find the four frantic, surviving missionaries holed up in their guesthouse. Listening to the heart-rending account of their horrendous experiences over the previous weeks, it seemed that virtually everyone stricken by Yambuku fever had died an agonizing death within a week. The nuns knew of only two survivors—one was Mbuzu ex-Sophie, wife of the head teacher, and the other was Sukato, a male nurse from the mission hospital.

Piot and his colleagues still had no clue how the virus spread or how long it could survive in the environment. So before turning in for the night, as a precaution, they fumigated a mission school classroom and mopped the floor with bleach before sleeping on the bare boards. They had just three or four days before returning to Kinshasa and their brief was clear. They had to identify and take blood samples from Yambuku fever sufferers, and from anyone who had recovered, for virus testing. Also, they were to assess the extent of the outbreak and determine how active it remained. To work out how the virus was transmitted, where it came from, and the length of the incubation period they had to ask innumerable questions about sufferers' everyday lives. First, questions about recent travel or contact with travellers or traders, contact with wild animals, or consumption of unusual food or drink. Then when, where, and from whom the sick and their families thought they had acquired the infection. All this was a lot to ask traumatized and suspicious villagers. In return the team hoped to do what they could to prevent further virus spread and to relieve suffering. But with no effective treatment on offer, they were unsure how cooperative the villagers would be.

The next day the group got to work early. Four Land Rovers were available and so they split into four groups and set off to survey the surrounding villages. In each village—small collections of mud huts topped by banana-leaf roofs—they first reported to the village chief and elders with whom they were obliged to share a drink of *arak*—crudely distilled banana alcohol—from a single plastic cup. Piot and his group saw eight sick people that first morning, one of whom was so ill that he actually died while they were taking blood from his moribund wife lying beside him. Almost all villages reported at least one death, but the team were encouraged to find several where presently there were no sick people, and some people who claimed to have recovered from the disease. Mostly these lucky ones attributed their recovery to the services of the *nganga kisi*—the local sorcerer or herbalist. But, interestingly, the survivors seemed to have had a mild form of the disease with no haemorrhagic symptoms. Of course, their symptoms could have been caused by a variety of other diseases and it was vital to distinguish these from Yambuku fever. The only way to do so was to take a blood sample to test for antibodies against Yambuku fever virus. Fortunately, Sister Marcella accompanied the team on these visits and encouraged villagers to cooperate, but the downside of her presence was that it discouraged patients from admitting to visiting the *nganga kisi* rather than seeking help at the mission clinic.

Piot wrote a first-hand account of his experiences in Yambuku in his memoir published in 2012.[4] In it he describes these first few harrowing days in Yambuku:

> For the next two days we toured villages every morning, taking blood where we could, jotting down every potentially telling detail and piece of data we could muster. We saw patients with blood crusting around their mouths or oozing from their swollen gums. They bled from their ears and nose and from their rectum and vagina; they were intensely lethargic, drained of force.[5]

They followed human chains of infection to unravel the spread of the virus through Yambuku and surrounding villages, documenting many distressing family tragedies like this one taken from Piot's account:

> We heard of entire families who had been wiped out by the swift-moving virus. In one case, a woman in Yambuku had died days after giving birth, swiftly followed by her newborn. Her thirteen-year-old daughter, who had traveled to Yambuku to take charge of the child, fell ill once she returned to her home village and died days later; followed by her uncle's wife, who had cared for her; then her uncle; and then another female relative who had come to care for him. This extremely virulent interhuman transmission was frightening'.[6]

Frightening certainly, but it was just this kind of story that revealed the virus's mode of transmission. Picking off one relative at a time as in this family is typical of a virus spread by close person-to-person contact. If, on the other hand, the virus, like 'flu and measles viruses, spread through the air, or, like yellow fever virus, via an insect vector, it would have caused a much larger epidemic that would have been far more difficult to control without specific drugs or vaccines.

The team met in the evenings to compare notes. To construct a picture of the outbreak they made a simple graph with numbers of new cases plotted against time. To their intense relief this showed that the peak of the outbreak had passed. With a definite recent decline in new cases in the Yambuku area, they hoped the worst was over. They found that health care workers at the mission hospital were at high risk of catching the disease; unsurprising as they took no precautions to protect themselves, with the highly infectious virus later being shown to be present in blood and all other bodily fluids. But the data also identified some unexpected links between the virus and its victims. First, almost every one of the early cases had attended the Yambuku mission hospital before they developed Yambuku fever. And, intriguingly, these cases consisted of twice as many women as men. Further scrutiny of the nuns' hospital and clinic ledgers revealed that most of the deceased women had been pregnant and had attended an antenatal clinic at the mission hospital. But still, the way in which they had all contracted the virus remained a mystery until the team questioned the surviving nuns. They admitted that they only had five glass syringes in total for use in the clinic. These were boiled every morning and then re-used throughout the day, perhaps with a quick rinse in sterile water between patients. Also, at the antenatal clinic, all pregnant women, healthy or not, were given injections of vitamin B and calcium gluconate at each visit. The latter is of no medical benefit.

Clearly this was the root of the problem—the school head teacher, now recognized as patient zero, the index case for this outbreak, had gone to the mission hospital with non-specific symptoms for which the nuns gave him an injection of chloroquine for malaria. Then, following their usual practice, they continued to use the same unsterile syringe and needle to deliver drugs to other patients throughout the day, including many antenatal patients attending for their vitamin injections. Most of these women and their newborns succumbed to Yambuku fever, so bringing the proportion of women amongst the victims to 70%.

The second strong risk factor identified was attending a funeral of a victim. And again the explanation was unexpected. Among the people of Central Africa funerals are very important occasions, during which the deceased's spirit is freed to join his/her ancestors' spirits in the forest. Generally, the extended family and friends come from miles around to join villagers in the ceremonies and celebrations, which may continue for several days. During the outbreak both travelling and attending large gatherings inevitably encouraged spread of the virus, but more important seemed to be close contact with the corpse itself. Local custom dictated that before burial family members must wash the body thoroughly, including the mouth and other orifices. Given that the body of an Ebola victim is often covered in blood, faeces, and vomit, all of which contain the active virus, it is no wonder that those involved are at very high risk of becoming infected.

Just one cluster of cases mystified the team because they were unable to trace a link between it and any other cases. Sufferers had attended neither a hospital nor a funeral, but the mystery was solved when one survivor revealed the whole story. Apparently a young, pregnant woman developed a severe headache after returning from the antenatal clinic at Yambuku mission hospital. She called the *nganga kisi*, who treated her by scarification—making multiple, shallow cuts across her forehead with a knife. He then treated several other perfectly healthy women in the village in the same way, and with the same knife, to prevent them also suffering from a headache.

As mentioned earlier, in addition to collecting data, the team were keen to do what they could for the sick and dying. Without any specific treatment the only option was to try infusing sufferers with antibodies from the blood of survivors in the hope of saving their lives. But this is a difficult task at the best of times. Obtaining antibodies requires taking large volumes of blood as well as using a sophisticated plasmapheresis machine to separate the blood plasma containing antibodies from other blood components. The equipment was only available in Kinshasa, and so the group had to persuade the two known survivors, Sophie and Sukato, to make the trip to the capital. This was asking a lot since neither had even visited Bumba before let alone Kinshasa. But Sophie had lost two of her eight children to the disease as well as her husband and so, despite her grieving, she was keen to help, and eventually both she and Sukato agreed to go.

The subgroup had instructions to return to Kinshasa with their precious blood samples and so after four days in Yambuku they drove to Bumba accompanied by the fearful Sophie and Sukato. Their plane, which eventually arrived four days late, delivered them safely to the capital on October 27 when the two convalescents were taken to Clinique Ngaliema to have their blood tested for antibodies against the Yambuku fever virus.

* * *

Piot soon returned to Yambuku to continue the investigation and prepare for the arrival of the Commission, but by the time the whole team reached the mission at the beginning of November the outbreak was over. Nevertheless, they had important work to do.

Thankfully, they had already achieved their top priority by preventing an outbreak in Kinshasa. They then spent time in the capital city preparing for the task ahead. Under stressful conditions, and in one of the poorest countries in the world, it was no easy task to train personnel and organize supplies, medical equipment, and sophisticated laboratory facilities, all to be transported to the remote village of Yambuku. To quote from their report to WHO, the circumstances 'at times seemed to us those of a small war'.[7]

Although the advance party's quick survey provided a clear snapshot of the outbreak in the Bumba Zone, this was never intended to be a scientific study. The full Commission arrived complete with vehicles, trained staff, ample food supplies, a generator, and a portable, high-containment laboratory for virus antibody testing, which they set up at the mission hospital. They then set about investigating the extent of the outbreak and identifying any active and convalescent cases, defining the clinical and epidemiological features of the disease and searching for the origin of the virus. First they had to devise a case definition for the haemorrhagic fever so that all surveillance teams were investigating the same disease. In view of the non-specific nature of most of the symptoms, and without backup laboratory virus testing, this was not easy. But eventually they defined a 'probable case' as: 'a person living in the epidemic area who died after one or more days with two or more of the following symptoms and signs: headache, fever, abdominal pain, nausea, and/or vomiting and bleeding. The patient must have, within the preceding three weeks, received an injection or had contact with a probable or proven case, the illness not having been otherwise diagnosed on clinical grounds.'[8]

An epidemiological survey was initiated using ten surveillance teams that had been recruited and trained for the job in Kinshasa.

All teams comprised four people, a team leader—a doctor or nurse—two nurses, and a driver with a four-wheel-drive vehicle. Teams were given a planned, individual route in the epidemic zone extending up to 200km from Yambuku. Each route included up to fifty-five villages, which were all visited on three occasions. In every village the teams' task was to conduct a house-to-house survey recording all family members, numbers of active and past cases, deaths, and survivors. Of course, most of those who had suffered from the disease were now dead, so the teams interviewed close relatives and then asked the same questions of two or three control subjects of the same age and sex from the same village who had not suffered from Yambuku fever. Blood samples were collected from all suspected cases, recovered cases, and controls. It was a massive undertaking which took almost a month to complete.

The surveillance teams eventually visited 550 villages and interviewed around 238,000 members of 34,000 families. Some 231 probable cases of Yambuku fever were identified but none was confirmed by antibody testing. By the end of November it was clear that the last case had died on November 5 in Bongulu II village, 30km east of Yambuku. On December 16 quarantine was lifted in the Bumba Zone.

The results of this larger study broadly agreed with the findings of the advance subgroup. The index case for the outbreak in Yambuku was confirmed as Mabalo Lokela, the head teacher from the mission school, who first became ill on August 26. So the important question to answer was: where did he catch the virus? Either he acquired it from an infected person or from an unknown animal source. Thus the details of the trip he took just prior to his illness became all important. Between August 10 and 22, 1976, Lokela had toured the Mobaye-Bongo Zone in the north east of the Equateur Region with six other men. On August 22 he bought fresh and smoked antelope and monkey meat from a road-side stall 50km north of Yambuku. On his return he and his family stewed and ate the antelope meat but did not eat the monkey meat.

The Commissioners knew that an outbreak of a similar haemorrhagic fever had been ongoing in southern Sudan since June 1976, centred on the townships of Nzara and Maridi near the border with DRC some 724km (450 miles) from Yambuku (Figure 1). In early November, just as the Commission was assembling, they heard that this outbreak was caused by a virus identical to that isolated from the dead nuns from Yambuku. So, naturally, they considered the possibility that these two outbreaks were linked. Two surveillance teams were air-lifted to northeast Zaire to undertake an intensive search for active cases between the Bumba Zone and the Sudanese border. Having travelled over 5,000km in the area, they failed to find any evidence of the disease that might form a link between the two outbreaks. However, they did ascertain that truckloads of people regularly travelled between southwest Sudan and Bumba, a journey of around four days. This suggested that someone incubating the virus could have reached Yambuku before falling ill, but in the end they were unable to firmly establish the origin of the outbreak in Yambuku. They thought that the most likely explanation was that the virus was brought from southern Sudan to Yambuku by a person rather than being introduced directly into the Yambuku population from an unknown animal host. In addition, Lokela could have encountered an infectious person during his trip north or he could have been infected from the bush meat he brought home with him. This uncertainty was resolved several years later when more sophisticated virus genome sequencing techniques became available that could distinguish between individual virus strains (see Chapter 2).

The surveillance confirmed that Yambuku mission hospital was the epicentre of the whole outbreak, because of the re-use of virus-contaminated syringes and needles. Receiving an injection at the hospital was the commonest risk factor for developing Yambuku fever during the first four weeks of the epidemic, with eighty-five sufferers being recipients of one or more injections at the Yambuku clinic. Thereafter the virus spread from person to person via close contact with bodily fluids. Comparing those who acquired the disease exclusively by injection with those infected by close contact with a case showed that the injection route was particularly lethal. The mean incubation period for the injection-acquired group was shorter (6.3 days versus 9.5 days), and the death rate was higher—100% versus the overall 88%. So the Commission concluded that closure of the mission hospital at the beginning of October had hastened the end of the outbreak by preventing villagers acquiring the virus from contaminated injection equipment. Interestingly, in contrast to the preliminary study, this large, controlled study did not find mere attendance at the funeral of an Ebola victim to be a significant risk factor for catching the disease. But if they had looked specifically at those involved in the funeral rites who actually touched the corpse they would most likely have uncovered this risk factor.

Plasmapheresis equipment arrived from Kinshasa on November 16 and was set up in the Yambuku mission hospital. Both Sophie and Sukato donated antibodies, and, as we will see in Chapter 2, within a month one of these donations was urgently required in the UK.

The epidemiological survey identified five of 442 people from four villages unaffected by the 1976 outbreak of Yambuku fever who, nevertheless, tested positive for virus antibodies. This suggested that the virus had infected people in the area before, although the finding may have been misleading as in those days Ebola testing was not always reliable. Be that as it may, the virus disappeared completely after the Yambuku outbreak and so the Commission were convinced that between outbreaks it hid in an animal reservoir. They searched for the virus in a large number of wild and domestic species from affected villages and the surrounding forest. These included bedbugs, mosquitoes, pigs, cows, a variety of bats, rats, monkeys, squirrels, and duikers, but they failed to recover the virus from any of these animals. And so the question of where the virus hides between outbreaks in humans remained unanswered.

Before the Commissioners left Zaire on December 22, 1976, they formulated a set of guidelines on how to deal with another outbreak of Yambuku fever. Their recommendations to the Zairian Government were that the country should:

- maintain active surveillance for, and increase awareness of, acute haemorrhagic fevers;
- distribute information to health care workers on acute haemorrhagic fevers and the proper methods for sterilizing injection equipment; and
- keep an up-to-date list of experienced Zairian experts and basic stocks of protective clothing and plasma from immune donors.[9]

Commission members also set about naming this new, lethal virus that had just killed 88% of the 318 people it infected. Traditionally, viruses were named after the town, city, or area from which they were first isolated, like Spanish or Hong Kong 'flu. But in this case, the Commissioners felt that the name 'Yambuku virus' would further stigmatize a village already devastated by its effects. So they thought it more appropriate to name the virus after the nearby Ebola River, a branch of the mighty Congo River; Ebola meaning 'black' in Lingala.

2

Ebola

The Virus and the Disease

The Prince Leopold Institute of Tropical Medicine in Belgium has been the alma mater of Belgian doctors working in the tropics since the early 1900s. Stefaan Pattyn, Professor of Micro biology at the Institute in the 1970s, had previously worked in Zaire, and so it was not unusual for him to help out with diagnostic problems from the country. But the package that arrived in his laboratory on September 29, 1976, was indeed unusual. It was, in fact, a blue plastic Thermos flask which, as we discovered in Chapter 1, was sent by Dr Jacque Courteille and contained blood samples from the Yambuku nun taken when she was severely ill with a haemorrhagic fever of unknown cause in Clinique Ngaliema in Kinshasa. With extraordinary disregard for the health and safety regulations that now seem to dominate our lives, the Thermos flask had been carried as hand luggage by a passenger travelling to Belgium on a scheduled passenger flight from Kinshasa! When the Thermos arrived in the laboratory the staff only knew that it contained 'samples of blood from an unusual epidemic that seemed to be stirring in the distant Equateur Region [of Zaire], along the river Congo', and that the working hypothesis for the epidemic was 'yellow fever with hemorrhagic manifestations'.[1]

In his book[2] Peter Piot describes how he and his colleagues in Pattyn's laboratory, without a thought for their own safety, or that of others, open the Thermos on the bench with just cotton lab coats and latex gloves for protection. Inside they find two tiny test tubes floating in melting ice. And to make matters worse, one of the tubes is broken; its contents mixing freely with the ice and water to form a lethal brew. Nothing daunted, they extract the intact tube of blood, simply labelled 'no. 718', and proceed to test the contents for antibodies against a variety of microbes that cause tropical fevers including yellow fever, typhoid fever, and another African viral haemorrhagic fever called Lassa fever. When all these tests give negative results, the group begin to think that any antibodies in the sample must have been destroyed as it thawed during the journey from Kinshasa. But, in order to isolate any viruses that might be present, they also inject sample no. 718 into tubes containing growing monkey cells and into the brains of adult and newborn mice—all places where viruses like to grow. It is these tests that come up trumps. On October 4 one adult mouse dies and another succumbs on October 5. Then all the newborn mice die as well—a sure sign of a lethal virus growing in their brains. The laboratory at the Institute is certainly not equipped for handling such a potentially dangerous virus, but even with these warning signs the team do not stop work on the sample or even implement any extra safety precautions. Excitement takes hold, and when the cultured cells also begin to die, indicating that they too are infected with a virus, Piot and colleagues continue to handle the infected material on the open bench. But by this time officials at WHO have got wind of what they are up to. They instruct Pattyn to send all the material to the British Army High Security Laboratory at Porton Down, Wiltshire, UK—the nearest of just three laboratories in the Western world in the 1970s that had the biohazard level 4 (category 4) containment facilities required for handling haemorrhagic fever viruses safely (the other two being CDC in Atlanta, and the US Army Biological Warfare Laboratory at Fort Detrick in Maryland).

A furious Pattyn complies with WHO's orders, but only partially. He tells the team to send the remains of sample no. 718 to Porton Down but to retain some of the dying cell cultures and ailing mice in the laboratory. They do so, and by October 12 the cells are ready to process for inspection under an electron microscope (EM). This type of microscope has a magnification power up to 1,000 times that of a conventional light microscope and is the only way to actually visualize anything as tiny as a virus, which would be between 20 and 400 nanometres (nm) in size (1nm is 0.000000001m). The Institute does not own such a large and expensive piece of equipment so the team take the prepared samples to an EM facility at Antwerp University Hospital where a friendly expert agrees to help. As he sits in the darkened EM room, the beam of electrons hits the specimen, illuminating and magnifying it. He peers at the EM screen and snaps a photo of the resulting image. Back at the Institute the team have a few anxious hours to wait before he reappears with the photo. It shows a long thread-like structure that looks nothing like yellow fever virus or any other traditional virus known at the time (Figure 2). But Pattyn knows exactly what it looks like, and the knowledge scares him. He immediately stops the experiments and sends all remaining material to Karl Johnson, the haemorrhagic fever expert in the Virology Division at CDC, Atlanta.

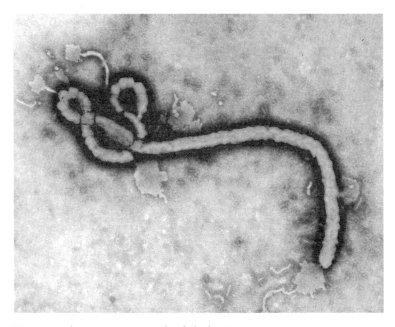

Figure 2 Electron micrograph of Ebola virus.

The thread-like virus in the EM photo reminded Pattyn of the dreaded Marburg virus that first reared its head in August 1967, causing an outbreak of haemorrhagic fever. This involved thirty-one cases occurring simultaneously in Marburg (twenty-three cases) and Frankfurt (six cases), in Germany, and in Belgrade, the capital of Yugoslavia (two cases). The link between the three towns was immediately obvious because all the initial sufferers were employed in laboratories of Behringwerke, a pharmaceutical company owned at the time by Hoechst. The common factor in the affected laboratories was grivet monkey cells that were being used to grow polio virus for vaccine development. A consignment of live grivet monkeys (*Cercopithecus aethiops*) had recently arrived from Uganda when twenty-five laboratory staff became unwell.

Exactly like the disease experienced in the Yambuku Ebola outbreak, the illness began suddenly with fever, headache, and malaise,
progressed to abdominal pain, diarrhoea, and vomiting and, in
most cases, both internal and external bleeding. Haemorrhagic
fever was diagnosed and a virus was quickly isolated from the
patients' blood. This was described in the scientific publication
that documented the outbreak as: 'most unusual. It differs in size
and shape from most known viruses. The mean length is 665nm'.[3]
The source of the virus was traced to the grivet monkeys, with
human infection occurring through handling the animals' blood
and organs without adequate protection. Five more people caught
the virus by contact with blood from the sufferers, and a further
case occurred three months later—the wife of a patient who
apparently acquired the virus from her husband by sexual transmission. Seven of the twenty-five who were infected by handling
material from sick animals died of the disease, while all the others
recovered, giving an overall fatality rate of 25%. Only three more
cases of Marburg are known to have occurred prior to the 1976
Yambuku Ebola outbreak; all in a single episode in South Africa in
1975. A young man developed the disease in Johannesburg, South
Africa, after spending several weeks touring in Rhodesia (now
called Zimbabwe). He died of the disease but his female compan-
ion who caught the virus from him, and a nurse who caught it
from her, both survived.[4]

Pattyn clearly knows about these two Marburg outbreaks and
so the questions that he and his colleagues ask themselves as they
stare at the EM image of the new virus on that day in October 1976
are: is Yambuku fever actually Marburg haemorrhagic fever? Or is
it caused by a related and equally lethal virus? When the excitement dies down the Belgian team decide to head for Kinshasa to

join the International Commission in investigating the Yambuku outbreak.

*   *   *

When sample no. 718 sent by Pattyn arrived at Porton Down, staff repeated the same tests as the Belgian team had set up, inoculating the blood sample into laboratory animals, this time including young guinea pigs, and cultured monkey cells. Unknown to Pattyn, they sent part of the sample direct to Johnson at CDC. So, in fact, all three teams, Belgian, British, and American, isolated the same thread-like virus resembling Marburg virus from the dead nun's blood. Additionally, at Porton Down they had received specimens from the ongoing haemorrhagic fever outbreak centred on the towns of Nzara and Maridi in Sudan from which they also isolated a Marburg-like virus. But tests to determine whether these viruses were actually Marburg virus or a different, but related, virus could only be performed at CDC where Johnson had stored Marburg virus and immune sera from patients who had recovered from the 1967 and 1975 Marburg outbreaks. Using these reagents he demonstrated conclusively that the Yambuku and Sudan virus isolates were a new and unique virus. All subsequently agreed on the name suggested by the International Commissioners in Yambuku—Ebola virus—and the disease it causes officially became Ebola haemorrhagic fever.[5]

Isolation of a new and very unusual virus was exciting, but then things took a very serious turn at Porton Down. Despite the fact that staff had followed all the advised precautions to protect themselves, the unthinkable happened—someone caught Ebola.[6] On November 5, 1976, virology technician Geoff Platt, dressed in full protective clothing, was injecting mashed-up liver from an infected guinea pig into an uninfected animal when he accidentally pricked his thumb through his rubber glove with the contaminated needle. He immediately removed the glove, immersed his thumb in a solution of chlorine sufficiently strong to kill all known viruses and then squeezed it hard. No blood emerged and no puncture wound could be seen in the thumb through a magnifying glass. Good news you might think, but six days later Platt began to feel unwell.

Just after midnight on November 11 Platt spiked a fever and then complained of abdominal pain and nausea. He was admitted to the High-Security Infectious Disease Unit at Coppetts Wood Hospital in London where he was placed in a negative-pressure plastic isolator. The results of virus testing on a blood sample taken on November 11 came through the next day bringing the worst possible news—characteristic thread-like Ebola virus particles were present in his blood. Over the next ten days Platt suffered the typical symptoms of Ebola with persistent fever, abdominal pain, loss of appetite, nausea, vomiting, diarrhoea, skin rash, sore throat, and severe lethargy.

Once the diagnosis of Ebola was confirmed, the doctors looking after Platt began to treat him with interferon, a natural product with general anti-viral properties. They continued this treatment for fourteen days in the hope that it would improve Platt's chances in the fight against the virus. They also sent an urgent request to DRC for immune plasma from a recovered Ebola sufferer. This arrived with remarkable speed and on November 13 Platt was infused with one unit of plasma taken from the Yambuku nurse, Sukato. He was given another unit, this time from Sudan, on November 16 when his symptoms were at their worst. The only additional treatment Platt received was intravenous fluids after he became dehydrated from diarrhoea and vomiting, and an antibiotic for a thrush infection in his throat. Fortunately, he showed no sign of bleeding into skin or mucous membranes and by November 20 his condition was improving; his temperature finally returning to normal on November 22. Unfortunately, it is impossible to judge from this single case whether or not the immune plasma and/or the interferon prevented the haemorrhagic manifestations of Ebola and thereby saved Platt's life. Not surprisingly, both during and after the acute illness Platt was subject to intense investigations. Daily blood samples were tested for Ebola virus, which was detectable for the first eight days of the illness. For reasons of safety other samples, such as faeces, urine, and throat swab, were not collected during the acute illness, but from day fourteen onwards all were negative. But in a completely unexpected finding, Platt's semen tested positive for Ebola virus at this stage and remained so for sixty-one days—long after the virus had disappeared from the blood. This finding, reminiscent of Marburg in 1969, first alerted doctors to the fact that Ebola was present in secretions and could remain in the body as a potential source of virus spread for several weeks after the patient had apparently recovered. From then on it was assumed that virus is present in all bodily fluids and that contact with these fluids is a common route of virus spread.

During the acute disease Platt suffered weight loss, hair loss, and anaemia, and was not completely well again until February 1977. Fortunately though, the virus did not spread to any member of his family or to the medical team—twenty-four nurses and five doctors—who cared for him during the acute illness.

* * *

Both Ebola and Marburg viruses belong to the family Filoviridae, meaning filamentous viruses and referring to the unique thread-like form of the virus particles. These particles vary in shape; sometimes they are branched or looped, adopting a circular, 6, or U shape (Figure 2). They are 80nm in diameter and anything up to 14,000nm in length—very long for a virus! The genetic material of filoviruses is RNA, and while there is only a single species of Marburg virus, there are five species of Ebola which differ genetically by at least 30% due to variations in their RNA sequence (that is, their genomes). These Ebola virus species also differ in the geographical location of the outbreaks and in the death rates they cause. Each species is named after its country or region of origin, thus the first Ebola virus isolated, that from sample no. 718 from Yambuku, is called *Zaire Ebola virus*.

Four of the five Ebola virus species cause highly lethal haemorrhagic fevers in humans, and the outbreaks they have caused were restricted to five countries in central Africa—DRC, Republic of Congo, Sudan, Uganda, and Gabon—until the 2014 outbreak struck in West Africa. Zaire Ebola is the most common and most lethal of the four species with a fatality rate up to 90%. Interestingly, thanks to major advances in molecular techniques since the 1970s, the virus recovered at Porton Down from the 1976 Ebola outbreak in southern Sudan is now known to differ sufficiently from Zaire Ebola to be designated a separate species—*Sudan Ebola virus*—with a fatality rate of around 40%. Thus the simultaneous outbreaks in Sudan and Zaire in 1976 were in fact derived from two separate introductions of Ebola to humans rather than a single introduction with virus spread from Sudan to Yambuku as the investigating Commission had speculated. Since that time these two viruses have caused most of the Ebola outbreaks in humans (Table 1).

In addition to humans, Ebola causes fatal haemorrhagic fever in non-human primates in the wild, particularly chimpanzees and

Table 1 Major Ebola virus disease outbreaks in chronological order

Date	Country	Ebola species	Case numbers	% Deaths
1976	DRC	Zaire*	318	88
1976	S. Sudan	Sudan	151	53
1979	S. Sudan	Sudan	34	65
1994	Gabon	Zaire	52	60
1995	DRC	Zaire**	315	81
1996	Gabon	Zaire	37	57
1996–97	Gabon	Zaire	47	74
2000–01	Uganda	Sudan	425	53
2001–02	Gabon	Zaire	65	82
2001–02	DRC	Zaire	43	75
2003	DRC	Zaire	35	83
2004	S. Sudan	Sudan	17	41
2007	Uganda	Bundibugyo	149	45
2009	DRC	Zaire	32	47
2012	Uganda	Sudan	11	36
2012	DRC	Bundibugyo	36	36
2013	Uganda	Sudan	6	50
2014	W Africa***	Zaire	28,637	40
2014	DRC	Zaire	66	74

* Yambuku
** Kikwit
*** Guinea, Sierra Leone, and Liberia

gorillas, and in some areas repeated outbreaks have devastated the populations of these endangered animals. The first proven outbreak affecting chimps was in Côte d'Ivoire, West Africa, in 1994. Several hundred chimps (*Pan troglodytes versus*) live in the country's Tai National Park, the largest area of tropical rain forest in West Africa, and in 1992 and 1994 one particular troop of chimps experienced outbreaks of a lethal, haemorrhagic disease.

This chimp troop was being closely monitored by scientists studying animal behaviour and on November 16, 1994, three of these scientists performed an autopsy on a recently deceased animal.[7] During the procedure they took few precautions against infection, and eight days later one of them, a 34-year-old, female, Swiss scientist, became unwell with fever, headache, chills, muscle aches, and a cough. She was admitted to hospital in Abidjan, the capital of Côte d'Ivoire, where she was treated for malaria. But when her fever did not abate and she developed vomiting, diarrhoea, and a skin rash as well as mental disturbances, she was repatriated to Switzerland.[8] Fortunately, she made a full recovery and no further cases occurred. Subsequently, a filovirus was isolated from blood samples taken during the acute phase of her illness and shown to be a new species of Ebola virus.[9] Tissues from a chimp that died in the outbreak also tested positive for Ebola, and this new species is now named *Tai Forest Ebola virus*. But the question of how and where the chimps acquired the virus remained unanswered.

The most recently isolated Ebola species is *Bundibugyo Ebola virus*, which first caused an outbreak in Bundibugyo District of western Uganda in 2007, with fifty-six laboratory confirmed cases. Interestingly, only a minority of cases (45%) developed the haemorrhagic symptoms that cause tissue damage and consequently the fatality rate was lower than for *Zaire Ebola virus* at around 40%.[10]

Studies undertaken in isolated communities in Gabon,[11] and among the Aka Pygmy population in Central African Republic[12] in areas where no Ebola outbreaks had been recorded, showed significant levels of immunity to Zaire Ebola, although once again the specificity of the Ebola tests used has been questioned. If true, this finding provides evidence of past infection in between 10 and 20% of inhabitants and suggests that Ebola is more common than was previously thought. Also, in this situation the virus must cause non-epidemic isolated infections that are non-haemorrhagic and non-fatal. In recognition of this and of data from other outbreaks of Zaire Ebola where the haemorrhagic disease was less common than in Yambuku, the official name of the disease the virus causes was changed from Ebola haemorrhagic fever to Ebola virus disease.

Reston species of Ebola virus is the exception to the general rules that filoviruses cause severe haemorrhagic fevers in humans and are restricted to tropical Africa. This virus was first isolated in 1990 from crab-eating macaques (*Macaca fascicularis*) which had been imported from the Philippines to a laboratory in Reston, Virginia, US, for experimental purposes. They quickly became ill and died of a haemorrhagic fever.[13] A new species of Ebola virus was isolated from them and called *Reston Ebola virus*. Of the 186 animal handlers tested for virus antibodies, twelve were positive, including four of five workers from the animal hospital.[14] One worker who cut himself while handling the liver of a dead, infected animal also had antibodies to the virus, but none of these workers became unwell. More recently there have been outbreaks of Reston Ebola in farmed pigs in the Philippines with virus spread to the pig farmers.[15] The infected farmers also remained healthy, so, fortunately, it seems that presently this Ebola virus is not a threat to humans.

* * *

Several types of viruses can cause haemorrhagic fevers, but none is as lethal as Ebola. These haemorrhagic fever viruses, including Lassa fever and yellow fever viruses, belong to different virus families, but share certain characteristics with Ebola. For instance, they all have RNA genomes and are animal viruses, which occasionally cause a so-called zoonotic infection in humans. Zoonotic viruses are primarily animal viruses that occasionally jump to humans causing a zoonotic infection, but they cannot survive in humans long term. This reliance on an animal host generally restricts human infection to the specific geographical area where the primary hosts live. It also means that outbreaks in humans occur sporadically and are very difficult to predict. As discussed in detail later, the identity of the primary host for Ebola is still subject to some uncertainty, but for most haemorrhagic fever viruses the animal host is well established. Lassa fever virus, for example, is endemic in West Africa because it is carried by the multimammate rat (*Mastomys natalensis*) that lives in this region. The virus is named after the town in Nigeria where the first known cases occurred when two missionaries died of the disease in 1969. While most sufferers are infected by direct contact with infected rats or their excreta, person-to-person transmission can occur through contact with a patient's bodily fluids. The disease is actually much more common than Ebola, with between 100,000 and 300,000 cases annually in West Africa, and although the mortality rate is lower, it still accounts for around 5,000 deaths every year.

As already noted, yellow fever virus also causes haemorrhagic fever, but only in around 10% of cases. The virus primarily circulates among several species of monkey in the rain forests of tropical and subtropical Africa and South America. It is spread among them by forest-living mosquitoes but occasionally jumps to humans via a bite from one of these virus-laden insects. This can then cause an epidemic among humans spread by *Aedes aegypti* mosquitoes, a species that tend to live alongside humans in the tropics and subtropics. There are an estimated 200,000 cases and 30,000 deaths annually from yellow fever, most of which occur in Africa.

* * *

Ebola virus is present at very high levels in the blood during an acute infection when its level directly correlates with severity of disease. The virus is also found to a lesser extent in all secretions and excretions including saliva, mucus, vomit, sweat, faeces, tears, and urine, with most spread occurring through contact with blood, faeces, and vomit. Importantly, infectious virus is also present in semen and breast milk where it can persist for several months after recovery. This virus can transmit via semen to sexual partners but transmission to breastfed babies via milk has not been formally proven. Since very few (probably 1–10) Ebola virus particles are required to infect a person, it is not surprising that this virus passes with such apparent ease from patient to health care workers and family members unaware of either the diagnosis or the danger. The virus can survive for a few hours on dry surfaces such as a door handle or work top, and for several days in blood and probably also in faeces and vomit. So although infection via environmental transmission has not been documented it remains a possibility.

Like all viruses, Ebola virus particles consist of a piece of genetic material, in this case RNA carrying only seven genes, surrounded by a protective covering. So a virus must enter a living cell and requisition its RNA- and protein-making machinery in order to reproduce. The new viruses so formed then spread throughout the body repeating this infectious cycle again and again in healthy cells in a battle that only ends when either the virus kills the host or the host's immune response eliminates the virus.

Since the layer of skin that completely covers the outer surface of our bodies has a superficial covering of dead cells, viruses cannot infect intact skin, but must find a way to reach the living cells beneath. For a virus like Ebola, which lurks unheeded on unwashed hands, this is usually achieved either through a small, even microscopic, skin cut or abrasion or by the carrier touching mucous membranes of the mouth, nose or eyes which are not protected by a layer of dead cells. Once in contact with living cells each virus must attach to a specific molecule on the cell surface in order to get inside. The identity of these molecules, known as receptors, differs between virus families, and their distribution determines the pattern of the disease that a particular virus causes. For example, it is well known that HIV (human immunodeficiency virus) uses CD4 as its receptor, a molecule that is mainly restricted to immune cells called helper T lymphocytes. So these are the cells that HIV infects and eventually wipes out altogether causing the fatal immune deficiency, AIDS (acquired immunodeficiency syndrome).

In contrast to HIV, Ebola virus can infect a large variety of cells including those of mucous membranes, the immune system, endothelial cells that line blood vessels as well as cells in the liver, spleen, lungs, and most other organs. In addition to human cells, the virus also infects cells of many other species, indicating that Ebola's cell receptor must be widespread in nature. But, mainly due to the bio-safety restrictions on working with Ebola in the laboratory, this receptor molecule (or molecules) has not been positively identified. Nevertheless, the Ebola virus-coded membrane glycoprotein, which protrudes from the surface of the virus as three spikes, acts as the molecule that is presumed to bind to its as yet unidentified cell receptor in order for the virus genome to gain entry into a cell. Blocking this interaction with antibodies against the Ebola glycoprotein prevents virus infection so this protein is the target of most potential Ebola vaccines (see Chapter 7).

On entering the body the first cells Ebola encounters are macrophages. These are immune scavenger cells that patrol the tissues, including skin and mucous membranes, and mop up any dead or alive foreign material, carrying it to lymph glands to be dealt with by other types of immune cells. By infecting these mobile cells, Ebola virus hitches a ride to lymph glands where it can then infect more immune cells. As millions of viruses are produced by these infected cells, they spill over into the blood stream and are carried to most of the other organs in the body.

The common feature of all viral haemorrhagic fevers is, of course, the bleeding. But this specific feature is preceded by several days of non-specific 'flu-like symptoms. After an incubation period of anything between two and twenty-one days, but most commonly four to ten days, Ebola virus disease starts abruptly with fever followed by head and muscle aches and severe fatigue. These symptoms are caused by the virus growing in immune cells in lymph glands and circulating in the blood, and, unsurprisingly, in tropical areas they are often diagnosed as malaria. Frequently it is only when anti-malaria treatment fails and the patient develops vomiting and diarrhoea and a skin rash some five to seven days later, accompanied in the worst cases by bleeding, that the true diagnosis is even suspected.

Initially bleeding is caused by virus targeting blood vessel endothelial cells, punching holes in the vessel lining that allows blood to leak into skin, mucous membranes, and tissues. This results in bruising, pin-point haemorrhages called petechiæ, and bleeding from around venepuncture sites. Blood oozing from mucous membranes manifests as bleeding gums, ears, nose, and into the whites of the eyes, while internal bleeding damages organs, particularly the liver and kidneys. Injury to liver cells then potentiates the bleeding by reducing their capacity to manufacture proteins required for blood clotting.

While bleeding has been a characteristic feature of fatal Ebola infection in several outbreaks, the blood loss it causes is not generally life threatening, the one exception being rare cases of massive gastrointestinal tract haemorrhage. Generally, it is the combination of vomiting, diarrhoea, and fluid loss through damaged blood vessels leading to dehydration and low blood pressure that is so dangerous in Ebola. If left uncorrected, this causes a downward spiral with metabolic disturbances, shock, kidney shutdown, multi-organ failure, and almost inevitable death. In untreated cases of haemorrhagic Ebola, death usually occurs between six and sixteen days from the start of the illness.

*   *   *

The immune response to any virus infection is composed of two, linked, phases; the innate phase, which is the first line of defence and is a non-specific host response engendered by all invading organisms. This is followed by a later, specific phase that directly targets the invading organism. The innate response is triggered by macrophages that, amoeba-like, engulf the invaders into a vacuole in their cell cytoplasm at their site of entry. The process of engulfing an organism does not harm the macrophage but stimulates it to release a series of chemical signals called cytokines. These attract a variety of other immune cells to the site of infection, causing local inflammation. This in turn initiates a cascade of cytokine release that is essential to orchestrate the specific phase of the immune response, which is mediated by antibody-producing, and virus-killing, lymphocytes.

Ebola virus paralyses the immune response, so enhancing its own growth and spread within the body. When the virus meets a macrophage at its site of entry in skin or mucous membranes it infects the macrophage before the cell has a chance to engulf the virus. The virus then sets about reproducing in, and killing, the macrophage, thereby crippling the innate phase of the immune response on day one of the infection. What's more, dying macrophages release an inappropriate flood of cytokines that kills off masses of lymphocytes, so paralysing the specific immune response as well.[16]

Because of the remoteness and unpredictability of Ebola outbreaks, most information on how the virus actually causes the symptoms of Ebola virus disease has been gleaned from studies on infected laboratory animal models. These studies revealed that severity of disease correlated with viral load (levels of virus in the blood) but the exact cause of the symptoms remained obscure. Then, in 2010, scientists from Gabon and France published the results of a study on blood samples obtained from fifty-six patients with acute Ebola disease caused by *Zaire Ebola virus* during outbreaks in Gabon and Republic of Congo between 1996 and 2005.[17] This was the largest study conducted on human Ebola disease at the time, including blood from fourteen survivors and forty-two non-survivors, and was aimed at pinpointing key differences between the immune response in fatal and non-fatal Ebola. Comparing levels of fifty different cytokines between these two groups, scientists found that non-survivors had incredibly high levels of the cytokines produced by macrophages in the innate phase of the immune response. These rose to peak levels two days before death, reaching up to 1,000 times higher than those found in healthy controls. This massive, uncontrolled cytokine release constitutes a so-called 'cytokine storm', which was completely absent in the survivor group. In contrast, levels of blood lymphocytes and the cytokines they normally produce were extremely low in non-survivors compared to those in survivors, presumably because the cells were wiped out by the cytokine storm produced by macrophages.

While moderately elevated cytokine levels during an acute infection, as seen in the survivor group in this study, are beneficial, the cytokine storm detected in all non-survivors would certainly contribute to the vascular collapse, multi-organ failure, and shock syndrome typical of fatal Ebola. The hope is that future studies of this kind will identify one or more defects in the immune response in fatal cases that, if prevented or corrected, would tip the balance in favour of survival.

* * *

Ever since the first known outbreaks of haemorrhagic fevers caused by Marburg and Ebola viruses in 1967 and 1976 respectively, scientists have assumed that these infections are zoonotic. Certainly the viruses could not survive long term in human populations, at least in the traditional African village setting, because they are so lethal to humans that they would soon run out of new hosts to infect. And since most viruses need to infect a continuous chain of susceptible hosts in order to survive, they would soon die out themselves. Scientists argue that only when the respective primary hosts are identified will it be possible to work out how to stop the sporadic spillover of these dangerous viruses into humans. It is most likely that the culprit hosts carry the viruses as silent infections, which do not cause disease but could easily be passed on to others, probably via blood and secretions, so that the viruses survive long term in these animal populations. So although in the 1967 outbreak of Marburg, virus clearly spread to humans from monkeys, the fact that these animals themselves were sick and dying made it very unlikely that they were the primary host of Marburg virus. At the time it was suspected that the monkeys either acquired the virus in Uganda where they were caught from the wild or that it jumped to them from other animal species that were housed alongside them during their journey from Africa to Europe. Similarly, we know that Ebola virus infects subhuman primates, but since the disease they suffer is severe and often fatal we can be sure that they, like humans, catch the virus from another animal source.

Over the years many concentrated efforts have been made to find the natural reservoir of filoviruses. For Marburg virus the breakthrough came in July 2007 when miners prospecting for gold and lead in Kitaka Cave in western Uganda came down with the disease. The cave houses a colony of Egyptian fruit bats (*Rousettus aegyptiacus*) numbering around 100,000 animals, and an investigating team from CDC captured over 1,000 of these bats to look for Marburg virus. They tested the animals for Marburg antibodies and used the highly sensitive polymerase chain reaction (PCR) method to detect tiny amounts of virus RNA. They found both Marburg antibodies and virus RNA in around 5% of these bats, which carried viruses that closely matched those isolated from the infected miners. Live virus was isolated from five infected animals, proving that they had an ongoing infection with the virus that jumped to the miners. Additionally, viruses from individual bats differed sufficiently from each other to suggest that Marburg virus had been circulating and evolving in this bat colony for a long time, thus indicating long-term virus carriage.[18] How Marburg virus jumps from bats to humans is still not entirely clear but since bats infected with Marburg in the laboratory have virus in their mouths, contamination of fruit is a likely possibility.[19]

Compared to the search for the primary host of Marburg virus, that of Ebola virus has not been nearly as easy to uncover. However, in 2005 a scientific paper was published which partially clarified the situation, the details of which are recounted in the following chapter.

*   *   *

It is no coincidence that in the 1970s when Ebola was first discovered, two of the only three laboratories in the Western world with category four facilities to handle dangerous viruses like Ebola were affiliated to the armed forces. Why? Because of the interest in using such viruses as lethal weapons. Similar laboratories in the former Soviet Union were also interested in 'weaponizing' deadly viruses. Indeed, accidental cases of Marburg virus disease occurred in staff at the Russian State Research Centre of Virology and Biotechnology in 1988 and 1990, one of which was fatal. During the cold war years (1947–91) scare stories intimated that Russian military scientists had created an Ebola virus that transmitted through the air, and even an Ebola/smallpox hybrid virus—lethal organisms that would certainly spread much faster and further than Ebola itself. But as the perceived threat of an East–West war diminished, research on potential biological weapons was wound down. In response to the United Nations Biological Weapons Convention, it had ended completely in the West by the mid-1970s. However, it re-emerged in 2001 after the 9/11 terrorist attack when both politicians and the armed forces in the US and Europe again saw bioterrorism as a real threat. The danger now was terrorists getting their hands on deadly microbes and so this time the aim was preparedness. Funds were made available for research into a number of deadly microbes and production of Ebola vaccines and effective therapies became a top priority. More category four laboratories were built and bio-defence funding for Ebola research rocketed. It is thanks to this sudden injection of cash that we know a fair bit about Ebola virus and the pathological processes underlying the disease it causes. Also, on a practical front, several prototype vaccines and anti-viral agents were in production when the largest ever Ebola epidemic hit West Africa in 2014 (see Chapter 7).

3

Ebola

The Years After Yambuku

When we left Yambuku, Zaire, at the end of Chapter 1, it was late 1976 and the first ever recorded Ebola outbreak was over. Members of the International Commission had completed their work and they were on their way home for Christmas. But after their departure it was far from business as usual in Yambuku and surrounding villages. The mystery illness, which struck over a period of just eight weeks, had killed suddenly and indiscriminately. Men, women, and children died a painful and gruesome death and there was nothing either the nuns at the mission hospital or traditional healers could do to stop it. Close to nine out of every ten of those infected died as, virtually overnight, Ebola created widows, widowers, and orphans. When the nightmare finally ended everyone was in mourning.

This was the shocked community in which David Heymann (a CDC Epidemic Intelligence Officer Trainee in 1976, and later Assistant Director of WHO), the only Commissioner to remain in Yambuku, found himself. Perhaps he was chosen to stay behind because he spoke fluent French, the official language of Zaire, but also he had been in Zaire for a shorter time than the other Commissioners. Back in October 1976 as the others set off for Zaire, CDC officials sent Heymann to Dallas, Texas. Here he collected a mobile isolation unit belonging to NASA and transported it back to the Air Force base in Atlanta. The 1960s and '70s was the era of moon exploration and the space race, and with astronauts regularly returning from the moon's alien environment, the American public had concerns about an invasion of moon bugs. So each time US astronauts splashed down in the Atlantic Ocean they were immediately transferred from the space capsule to this isolator, complete with filters to trap any extraterrestrial microbes! Regardless of the effectiveness of this manoeuvre, CDC now planned to use the equipment for a more present threat—a Commissioner contracting Ebola. If the worst should happen they would fly the isolator to Zaire and use it to repatriate the patient safely to the US.

Heymann remained in Yambuku for ten weeks, including Christmas 1976 and New Year 1977, staying at the mission alongside the few surviving Belgian nuns. It must have been a gloomy festive season with the nuns stunned by recent events and probably feeling very far from home. Nevertheless, with Heymann's assistance they reopened the mission hospital and he helped them to understand the importance of infection control and how to cope with future Ebola outbreaks. So the nuns carried on with their work, only later returning to Belgium for much needed recuperation.

Heymann's main remit in Yambuku was post-outbreak surveillance. This meant visiting each affected village to check for any new Ebola cases, testing family members of cases to uncover silent infections and searching out Ebola survivors. The latter were as rare as they were valuable; Heymann needed to persuade them to donate blood so that their antibodies could be used to treat Ebola victims in future outbreaks. In the post-Ebola weeks and months it must have required a very tactful and sympathetic approach to win the confidence and cooperation of these grieving people. Notwithstanding, twenty-six survivors were found, thirteen of whom agreed to donate antibodies. Overall they provided 201 units of convalescent plasma. These were placed in long-term storage and strategically located around the Continent as an insurance against future Ebola outbreaks in Africa.

Ebola did not return to Yambuku; in fact the virus completely disappeared—but not for long. It reappeared in June 1977, this time in Tandala, Zaire, some 325km west of Yambuku (see Figure 1). Again Heymann, who was by then working in Cameroon, was on hand to help out. When I met with Heymann in London in June 2015 he recounted how, as soon as he heard the news, he and a colleague drove for two days across Cameroon and Central African Republic on dirt tracks to reach Tandala. But this time, thanks to Tom Cairns, the American physician at Tandala mission hospital, Ebola was contained and no outbreak ensued.[1] The previous year Cairns had visited Yambuku at the height of the Ebola outbreak, so when a 9-year-old girl was admitted to his mission hospital suffering from a haemorrhagic fever he immediately knew what to do. Despite the hospital being poorly equipped, he implemented barrier nursing and placed her in a makeshift isolation ward where she died the following day. Ebola was found in her blood but Cairns' quick thinking prevented any transmission to hospital staff. No trail of infection could be uncovered in the girl's village, Bonduni, some 20km from the mission, and so, as in Yambuku, the origin of the virus remained a mystery. However, a survey of hospital admissions over the previous year uncovered one similar fatal illness in a 12-year-old girl in February 1977. Her younger sister also suffered from the disease at the time and survived. Heymann, Cairns, and colleagues tracked her down and found that she tested positive for Ebola antibodies although all other family members were negative.

Sporadic cases like these two girls suggested that the virus must be hiding somewhere in northwest Zaire and that it jumped to humans more frequently than was previously realized. To find out how common Ebola infection actually was, missionaries and mission hospital staff from the whole area, including Tandala, were tested for Ebola antibodies. Of the fifty-one tested just one turned up positive for Ebola antibodies—Dr Cairns. At this point Cairns recalled an interesting event. Back in May 1972, while performing an autopsy on a bible school student who had died from presumed haemorrhagic yellow fever, Cairns cut his finger. Twelve days later he became sick, suffering a severe illness. However, he did not develop any haemorrhagic symptoms and after ten days he began to recover. In retrospect this was clearly Ebola, which luckily did not spread further—not even to his wife, who nursed him throughout the illness. So Cairns can claim the dubious honour of being the first ever documented case of Ebola!

A similar survey of eight villages within a 40km radius of Tandala but with no history of Ebola outbreaks uncovered seventy-nine of 1,096 (7%) villagers with Ebola antibodies. This result reinforced the idea that the virus was lurking somewhere close by and from time to time it jumped from its unknown primary host to humans but did not necessarily cause either severe disease or an outbreak.[2]

* * *

Following the Tandala outbreak Ebola disappeared from DRC for seventeen years, and during that time only caused one small outbreak in Maridi, Sudan. Then, as detailed in Chapter 2, in late 1994 a scientist caught Ebola during an autopsy on a chimpanzee carcass found in the Tai Forest, Côte D'Ivoire. The animal had died of an undiagnosed haemorrhagic disease that was rife among chimps in the forest at the time. The identification of Ebola in the scientist and then in the chimps was the first indication that chimps were susceptible to Ebola. Also this was the first human case of Ebola in West Africa and the first isolation of the *Tai Forest Ebola virus*. Following this incident, over the periods 1994–96 and 2001–03, there was a series of Ebola outbreaks in humans in the rain forests of Ogooué-Ivindo Province of northeast Gabon spreading into bordering Republic of Congo in west central Africa.[3] These outbreaks were all linked to ongoing Ebola outbreaks in local primate populations, mainly affecting gorillas but also involving chimps. Duikers (*Cephalophus* spp), which are small forest antelopes (usually herbivores, they supplement their diet with carrion when available), were also affected, probably through contact with infected ape carcasses.[4] These outbreaks severely depleted the populations of already endangered primates. Scientists and local trackers estimated that thousands of animals died of Ebola in the region, and calculated the reduction in animal numbers after an outbreak in 2003 as 56% for gorillas, 89% for chimps, and 53% for duikers. While duikers, with their rapid reproductive cycle, may rebound fairly quickly from such an assault, there were concerns that a combination of fatal infection, hunting, poaching, and a slow reproductive cycle could spell eventual extinction of the apes in west central Africa.[5]

The simultaneous Ebola outbreaks in humans in Gabon and Republic of Congo targeted small, forest-living communities who survived mainly on bush meat. The outbreaks were usually preceded by increased numbers of animal carcasses being found in the forest by local villagers. The index cases were always hunters who had either caught and butchered a sick animal or butchered one found already dead. On occasions Ebola then spread from the hunters to their families and an outbreak ensued. The virus involved was always *Zaire Ebola* species but genetic analysis revealed that different virus strains were isolated from different forest locations. This indicated multiple Ebola introductions into primates in the area, suggesting that primates were in closer contact with Ebola's primary host than humans were. But, once again, the identity of this animal host remained unknown.

*   *   *

In the thirty-eight years between the first two simultaneous Ebola outbreaks in Sudan and Yambuku, Zaire, in 1976 and the unprecedented epidemic of 2014–16 in West Africa, there were twenty-four recorded human Ebola outbreaks in central and west central Africa with transmission from the index case to at least one other person. The most noted of these outbreaks are listed in Table 1 and their location is shown in Figure 3, with the largest being in Gulu District of Uganda, in the year 2000, with 425 cases and 224 deaths.[6] Death rates varied between outbreaks from approximately 40% to 90%, but a definite pattern could be detected in the causation of the outbreaks.

For an Ebola outbreak or epidemic to occur, several factors have to come together, each on its own being insufficient to allow the virus to spread. Heymann uses the Swiss cheese model[7] to explain the phenomenon: 'It's like trying to thread a pencil through several layers of Swiss cheese,' he says. 'In order to do this one hole in each piece must align so that the pencil can pass all the way through.' For

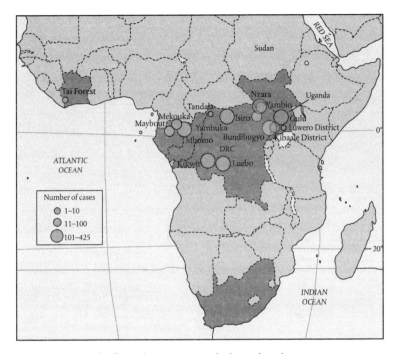

Figure 3 Map of Africa showing past Ebola outbreaks.

Ebola, the holes represent risk factors that must align simultaneously for an outbreak to occur. So what are these crucial risk
factors?

- First is emergence of Ebola virus from nature. Ebola outbreaks in
  humans prior to 2014 mainly occurred in rural communities in
  poor, central, and west central African countries (DRC, Gabon,
  Uganda, Sudan, and Republic of Congo), and each started with the
  virus jumping from a wild animal to a human.
- Second is amplification of virus transmission in poorly equipped
  health care facilities. Most outbreaks are kick-started by an index
  case being admitted to a hospital or health centre that lacks the

equipment and procedures necessary to prevent the virus spreading to health care workers and other patients. This is compounded by a lack of the necessary protective clothing as well as poorly trained health care workers looking after Ebola patients. Once a cluster of hospital staff is infected, they act as an unintentional link to the local community, carrying the virus to their homes and thereby amplifying transmission and triggering an outbreak.

• Third is poor disease surveillance combined with a lack of knowledge about Ebola. This leads to Ebola outbreaks initially being misdiagnosed as typhoid, yellow fever, or dysentery, and thus no effective precautions being taken to prevent the virus spreading. In this situation Ebola gets a head start as it spreads rapidly to surrounding communities.

• Finally, as mentioned earlier, funeral practices that involve touching the bodies of Ebola victims are a risk factor for Ebola spread in a community. In some areas local customs dictate that bodies are thoroughly washed by family members and close friends. The mouth and other orifices are flushed out while hair and nails may be kept as mementoes. Since bodies of Ebola victims are often contaminated with blood, vomit, and faeces, all of which contain live virus, this is clearly a hazard for contracting Ebola.

*   *   *

In an explosive Ebola outbreak such as that in Yambuku, it appears that the virus must be highly contagious, but in fact, when compared to airborne microbes such as measles and whooping cough (pertussis), this is not the case. Unlike these viruses, Ebola spreads by direct contact with blood or other bodily fluids from Ebola patients and in doing so establishes traceable chains of infection, mainly linking those who have been in closest contact with the patient—generally health care workers and family members. During an outbreak of any infectious disease, epidemiologists can predict its size and duration by calculating a key number called R_0. R_0 stands for 'case reproduction number', meaning the average number of new cases of the disease spawned by a single case. At the beginning of an epidemic R_0 is high as the microbe spreads through a largely non-immune population. Then, as the epidemic progresses and people in the affected community either die from the disease or recover and develop immunity to it, the value of R_0 begins to fall. The tipping point value for R_0 is one. If R_0 is above one then the infection rate is rising and an epidemic will ensue. In contrast, when R_0 falls below one then the infection rate is falling and the epidemic is coming under control. But although at this stage the worst might be over, new cases may continue to appear for a while to come, particularly if the microbe has a long incubation period.

The value of R_0 for measles and whooping cough ranges from 12 to 18, the highest for any acute infectious disease. Compared to this, R_0 for Ebola in a rural setting is just a modest 1.5–2.5, exemplifying the way Ebola typically only jumps from patient to carer forming an almost linear transmission chain. This is well illustrated by the following quote taken from the WHO Study Team Report on the outbreak in Sudan in 1976, which began in a cloth factory in the town of Nzara and subsequently spread to the town of Maridi. Forty-eight Ebola cases, including twenty-seven deaths, could be attributed to the infection of an extrovert character called PG:

The first identifiable case was YG, a storekeeper in the factory who became ill on 27 June 1976. He was nursed by his brother, who in turn became ill on 13 July. A second storekeeper, BZ, who worked alongside YG, was admitted to Nzara hospital on 12 July and died on 14 July. Soon afterwards his wife became ill and died at home on 19 July...The third man from the factory to fall sick was PG, who was employed in the cloth room beside the store where YG and BZ worked. PG became sick on or around 18 July and was admitted to Nzara hospital on 24 July; he died on 27 July...PG was a bachelor, who lived close to a shop belonging to a general merchant, MA. PG was reportedly an ebullient character, known to almost everyone in the area and he was closely associated with the merchant's family and employees. He was particularly friendly with two brothers, Samir S and Sallah S, who were staying in the merchant's household...During PG's illness he was visited by many people including two women, HW and CB, who nursed him before he was admitted to hospital.

Samir S became ill on 26 July and after a few days in Nzara he travelled with his brother Sallah, to Maridi on 6 August. There he became so ill that he was admitted to Maridi hospital on 7 August where he died on 17 August. Sallah helped to care for Samir in Maridi hospital and then returned to Nzara on 18 August, when he too began to feel ill. Meanwhile in Nzara four close contacts of PG—the two women HW and CB, together with SU, another cotton factory employee and close friend of PG, and RJ a nurse at Nzara hospital—had become ill and died of the disease. They in turn infected several others who had nursed them during their illnesses at home. Sallah arrived in Nzara on 18 August and was so ill the following day that he was visited by a hospital nurse, AI, who administered chloroquine and antibiotic injections. Sallah and one of the merchant's sons died later in the same house from the disease. The nurse, AI, fell ill on 24 August and was eventually taken to Maridi hospital where he died on 3 September. The merchant, MA, became ill on 21 August and went for treatment to Omdurman [a large city close to Khartoum, Sudan], travelling by road to Juba [capital of Sudan], and thence by plane to Khartoum. He died in Omdurman hospital on 30 August. Shortly after he left

Nzara, several of his family and employees also contracted the same illness.[8]

*   *   *

Despite all the inadequacies in disease surveillance and health care facilities that predispose to Ebola outbreaks in small, isolated, rural communities in central and west central Africa, because of Ebola's low R_0 value, these outbreaks are often self-limiting as the virus claims so many victims that it simply cannot maintain its chains of infection. And even if an outbreak does not die out spontaneously, once the diagnosis is clear and help arrives, it is generally fairly easily controlled by implementing the necessary precautions.

The large Ebola outbreak in Kikwit, Zaire, in 1995, initially epitomized all the defects and failures outlined above. In 1995, Zaire was in turmoil. After thirty years of corrupt and dictatorial rule by President Mobutu, the country was bankrupt and on the brink of civil war. The public sector was crumbling through total neglect and all over this vast country the devastating effects on health care, education, transport, and communications were all too apparent. Kikwit, a town with a population of around 200,000, was no exception. Situated on the banks of the Kwilu River some 475km—seven hours by (very bad) road—from Kinshasa (see Figure 1), the town's economy, such as it was, was based on subsistence farming, hunting, and fishing, with most people depending on the surrounding countryside for food. In 1995 the town had two hospitals, Kikwit General Hospital and Kikwit Maternity Hospital II, both in a state of neglect. It was among the staff of the latter hospital that an outbreak of Ebola, at first diagnosed as 'diarhee rouge' (bloody diarrhoea or epidemic dysentery), became apparent in early April of that year. At the end of April another cluster of cases occurred, this time among operating theatre staff at the General Hospital. This was thought to be a consequence of a sick laboratory technician from the Maternity Hospital being transferred to the General Hospital with suspected typhoid-associated bowel perforation (which was retrospectively diagnosed as Ebola). He underwent an abdominal operation performed by a surgical team with very little protective clothing—even latex gloves were in short supply. No bowel perforation was found and as his condition rapidly worsened another abdominal operation was undertaken at which massive intra-abdominal bleeding was noted. He died three days later. Fourteen hospital staff caught Ebola as a result of this incident including doctors, nurses, and two Italian missionaries.

By the time local experts arrived in Kikwit to investigate the outbreak at the beginning of May, long chains of infection had been established and the epidemic was widespread and out of control.[9] On May 4, in an attempt to control the infection, all hospitals, laboratories, health centres, and schools in Kikwit and the surrounding area were closed and suspected Ebola patients were confined to a quarantine ward in the General Hospital. But with no protective clothing, running water, electricity, toilet facilities, or food provision in the ward, isolation was impossible and so the control measure had little effect.[10]

Jean-Jacques Muyembe-Tamfum, at the time Zairian Minister of Health and a veteran of Ebola outbreaks, was among the first on the scene. Muyembe's extraordinary rags-to-riches life story began in a village in the Bandundu region of Zaire where he grew up the son of a poor farmer. He was educated by Jesuits and sent to Lovanium University, Kinshasa, to study medicine. While there he developed an enduring interest in the horrifying tropical infectious diseases he saw all around him. After gaining a PhD from Leuven University in Belgium Muyembe returned to DRC in 1973 to forge a career in outbreak control, saving countless lives while civil war raged all around him.

Back in 1976, while a young professor of microbiology at Kinshasa University Medical School, Muyembe was the first expert to visit Yambuku during the early days of the outbreak and he later joined the investigating Commission. At first he thought the dreadful suffering he witnessed in Yambuku was caused by typhoid fever and took blood samples from the sick to test for the typhoid bacterium back in Kinshasa. He noted that the patients bled profusely from the venepuncture site, and later admitted that he had been fortunate to survive the experience: 'My fingers and hands were soiled with blood. I just used water and soap to wash it off...We had no protective equipment, we didn't even have chlorine. I was lucky, yes, very lucky'.[11] And the whole world was lucky too. Since those early days Muyembe has controlled many Ebola outbreaks in DRC that might otherwise have spread widely. For this reason Heymann aptly describes him as 'the real unsung hero of Ebola control'.

It was Muyembe who recognized the Kikwit outbreak as Ebola rather than dysentery. And once this was confirmed by specific tests at CDC on May 9, an International Commission arrived to manage the response, coordinated by Muyembe and Heymann (the latter now leading an AIDS research team at WHO). Unsurprisingly, at the start the Commission found their work in Kikwit extremely difficult. No public health system existed and so it had to be constructed *de novo* employing rapidly trained local volunteers, many of whom were medical students whose lectures had been suspended by the crisis. They carried out all surveillance operations including case-finding, contact-tracing, and retrospective case counting. But with no prior knowledge of Ebola among the local community, case-finding was often hindered, on the one hand by families concealing, or denying the existence of, sick members and on the other hand by the reporting of non-cases in the hope of some monetary benefit for the reporter. Surveillance was also severely hampered by a lack of communication and transportation. With no telephones in the area, the team relied on 'phonies'—short wave radios belonging to the twenty-three Catholic missions in the Kikwit Diocese—for up-to-date information on new and follow-up cases. Catholic missions also organized patient meals and the distribution of new equipment and provided vehicles and fuel while local OXFAM and Red Cross volunteers assisted with public health education. The Red Cross also provided transport of cases to hospital and of safely wrapped bodies to burial sites.

Muyembe proved invaluable in the health education programme which was challenging because of low levels of literacy (~55%), closed schools, no local mass media, and a language barrier between Commissioners and the local inhabitants. Crucially, he could actually speak to the people directly in their own language, so while educational messages were broadcast through megaphones in the streets of Kikwit, he called local district leaders and village chiefs and elders together to explain the outbreak in terms that they could relate to. He described Ebola sufferers as being full of evil spirits that caused the illness as they tried to escape from the body. He said that if a healthy person touched a sick person then the evil spirits would enter them. He also explained the presence of foreigners, which might otherwise have caused resentment, as being necessary because these spirits were so strong that he needed help to stop them from spreading. With regard to the sensitive issue of traditional funeral rites, outside intervention, including seizing bodies for safe burial, had, in the past, soured relationships between village chiefs and those trying to help. Understandably, such actions were seen as an attack on traditional burial practices, which injured the spirit of the dead. Muyembe again explained the problem in terms of evil spirits, which jump from the dead to the living at the touch of a finger. Although all bodies had to be sealed in plastic bags and buried by a trained team, his solution was to distribute protective equipment to family members so that they could participate safely in the funeral rites.[12] To prevent hand contact that might spread the virus Muyembe and Heymann invented the 'Ebola greeting' while in Kikwit—touching elbows instead of shaking hands.

All these measures eventually brought the Kikwit Ebola outbreak under control. When the surveillance teams had completed their work, it was clear that the number of cases in Kikwit peaked in May and the last patient died on July 16, 1995 (Figure 4). But because the virus had had the upper hand for thirteen weeks, the beginning of the outbreak was difficult to pinpoint. Early cases misdiagnosed as dysentery had been admitted to a variety of hospitals and clinics or died at home, making it hard to unravel the sequence of events leading back to the index case. Nevertheless, it eventually became clear that the outbreak actually began long before the cluster of cases at the Maternity Hospital in April 1995. It transpired that on January 6 patient GM, a 42-year-old charcoal maker who lived in Kikwit but worked in the forest some 15km away, was admitted to Kikwit General Hospital with a haemorrhagic illness from which he died on January 13. He directly

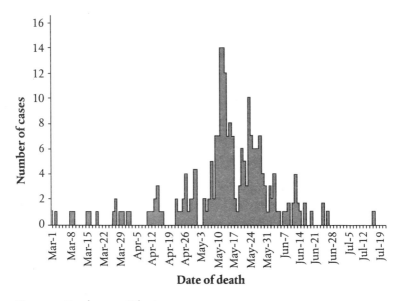

Figure 4 Fatal cases, Kikwit, 1995.

infected at least three members of his family and ten more cases occurred among his extended family in Kikwit and nearby villages over the following nine weeks. All thirteen cases were fatal. As no contact was identified for GM himself, and a link could be traced from him to the outbreak of so-called epidemic dysentery in Kikwit Maternity Hospital II beginning in mid-March, he was regarded as the index case for the whole outbreak.

The outbreak that began on January 6 was over by June 20, with just one further case occurring in mid-July. Overall there were 315 Ebola cases with an 81% fatality rate. 87% of cases were in Kikwit town but the virus also reached several villages within a 150km radius of Kikwit. One person who caught the virus in Kikwit travelled to Kinshasa before falling ill. He was admitted to a hospital where his illness was unrecognized and no precautions were taken to prevent virus transmission. Despite this no secondary Ebola cases occurred—a lucky escape for the capital city!

Of the 315 Ebola cases identified in the outbreak, 25% were health care workers. Fortunately, though, with just one exception, the arrival of protective clothing and implementation of barrier-nursing prevented further spread within hospitals and clinics. The one health care worker at the General Hospital who developed Ebola after the control measures were put in place wore protective clothing but mistakenly rubbed her eyes with soiled gloves.

Clearly, the Kikwit Ebola outbreak followed the familiar pattern of virus spread along chains of susceptible people, with an R_0 value of around 1.5. However, unexpectedly, the surveillance team uncovered two so-called super-spreaders. Super-spreaders are recognized in many epidemics, including those caused by 'flu, HIV, and SARS virus, as infected people who buck the trend by grossly exceeding the R_0 value for the particular microbe involved. So although R_0, the *average* number of cases derived from one case, in the Kikwit Ebola outbreak, was 1.5, these two victims far overstepped the mark. First was patient WB, a 29-year-old anaesthetist at the General Hospital who was a casualty of the fateful abdominal operation on the technician retrospectively diagnosed with Ebola. He was hospitalized for eight days in late April with raging, haemorrhagic Ebola before he died. He had many visitors during this time and thirty-eight subsequent Ebola cases reported contact with him while he was in hospital. The second super-spreader was a 45-year-old woman who was admitted to the Maternity Hospital with suspected dysentery but was later diagnosed with Ebola. After her death at the end of May her body was released to the family for burial. But despite the fact that by late May the community should have been aware of the dangers of Ebola, she was given a traditional funeral, including touching and washing the body. This resulted in twenty-one new cases of Ebola.

Other novel findings that emerged from the Kikwit outbreak included the realization that the incubation period for Ebola could be as long as twenty-one days, a possibility not entertained during the Yambuku outbreak. So the quarantine period for case contacts was extended to prevent the release of potentially infected people back into the community. Follow-up of Ebola survivors after recovery confirmed the previous finding of Ebola in semen samples. In this case, the virus persisted for up to ninety-one days after disease onset, although all other bodily fluids tested negative once the acute illness was over.[13] Additionally, several survivors developed uveitis, that is inflammation of the eyes, causing temporary visual disturbances, but thankfully no long-term problems ensued.[14]

* * *

In the nineteen years between the Yambuku and Kikwit outbreaks, times had changed in Zaire, and, with mounting political instability and impending bankruptcy, the memory of Ebola had faded. Disease surveillance in the Kikwit area was virtually non-existent and so the seriousness of the outbreak went unrecognized for thirteen weeks. At this stage a local District Health Officer notified national authorities of the outbreak but a further three weeks passed before the alarm was raised. In fact, it was the infection and death of most of the theatre staff in Kikwit General Hospital that finally brought a response from these authorities,[15] and even then there was a delay of another week while blood samples were sent via Belgium to CDC in the US for confirmation of the Ebola diagnosis. Then protective clothing and equipment necessary for barrier nursing of Ebola patients that had been stockpiled in strategic areas in DRC in 1976 were found to be out of date and had not been replenished. Yet more delays ensued while new supplies and equipment were purchased and shipped to the area.

The interval between the outbreaks in Yambuku and Sudan and that in Kikwit, had witnessed a complete revolution in global communications. While the 1976 Ebola outbreaks were dealt with in complete isolation, twenty years later members of the international media appeared on the scene in full force within two days of the International Commission's arrival; an event that took the Commissioners entirely by surprise. The presence of the press in Kikwit was a mixed blessing. On one hand, the vital work of the Ebola response teams was threatened by hordes of journalists and photographers in pursuit of a sensational story and/or a dramatic picture. They not only commandeered vehicles and occupied accommodation that was required for the response teams but also, by their intrusive insistence on filming Ebola victims, their grieving relatives, and their funerals without consent, they breached ethical standards and upset cultural sensitivities. Order was restored when Commissioners established daily press briefings and prearranged filming sessions. On the other hand, as news of the outbreak was beamed into millions of homes across the globe, money, supplies, and equipment were rapidly mobilized. WHO and international non-governmental organizations (NGOs) such as MSF, International Red Cross, and EPICentre, as well as individual physicians, virologists, and epidemiologists from national and international centres were alerted by the news coverage and came to help.

* * *

Following the Kikwit outbreak Muyembe and colleagues wrote: 'As long as the hygienic conditions remain substandard in many African hospitals and health care workers are unable to adhere to universal precautions to prevent the transmission of bloodborne infections, there is a risk of new EBO [Ebola] outbreaks in African cities.'[16] Nonetheless, the outbreak became a significant milestone in the history of Ebola management. It was the first to attract global attention and this in turn attracted global assistance. The resulting guidelines on the control of an Ebola outbreak served admirably until the 2014 Ebola epidemic in West Africa when, at least initially, they were not followed to the letter (see Chapter 4). In addition, many lessons were learned that had wider implications for infectious disease outbreaks throughout the developing world. These can be summarized as follows:[17]

- There was a pressing need for stronger public health practices in developing countries including disease detection, control, and prevention. This required training and skills development at a local level as well as the availability of essential supplies and provision of suitably staffed and equipped diagnostic laboratories.

- In recognizing the power of the international media in attracting public sympathy and resources for infectious disease control, the public health community should accommodate the needs of the press without detracting from their primary mission of controlling the outbreak as quickly as possible.

- WHO needed to act as the central authority for providing guidance for outbreak response teams and freely available, up-to-date information on current outbreaks for governments and the general public. The guidelines for coping with future Ebola outbreaks were in fact extremely simple and logical, consisting of three main imperatives: 1) isolation of patients with barrier nursing to protect health care workers; 2) tracing, quarantining, and monitoring all patient contacts (by regular measurement of body temperature); and 3) public engagement including addressing the sensitive issue of funeral customs in the particular region of the outbreak.

- Following the novel experience of NGOs responding to the Kikwit outbreak, international coordination was required in future outbreaks in order to use their unique skills and resources to maximum benefit. In response to this, WHO set up the Global Outbreak Alert and Response Network (later renamed the Global Alert and Response Network) with 120 partners worldwide to provide logistic support and training during infectious disease outbreaks.

- Finally, the Commission were aware that in the heat of an outbreak any attempt at research was often marginalized. For example, during the Kikwit Ebola outbreak convalescent blood had been used to treat some patients, but no clinical trial was undertaken and so no conclusions had been reached as to how effective this treatment was. Additionally, although antiviral agents were available, and despite the very high mortality rate, these drugs were not tested on Ebola victims. Thus this outbreak highlighted a need for scientific studies to be carried out in parallel with the provision of the best supportive care available. Only then could lessons be learned and applied in the next outbreak.

* * *

By the beginning of the twenty-first century, despite a great deal of work and many individual studies, the animal reservoir for Ebola virus in the wild remained elusive. Scientists knew that until this animal was identified Ebola outbreaks would continue to appear sporadically and unpredictably. Many observations over the years related Ebola outbreaks to bat infestations, but these associations remained anecdotal. In 2001–03, when Ebola outbreaks occurred simultaneously in humans, chimpanzees, and gorillas in Gabon and the Republic of Congo, some progress was finally made. A team of scientists from Gabon undertook trapping expeditions in the outbreak area, catching a total of 1,030 animals, including bats, birds, and small land mammals, in close proximity to dead gorillas and chimps. They tested for antibodies and used the highly sensitive PCR test to detect viral RNA in the animals' organs. Three different species of fruit bats came up positive in both tests and the PCR result indicated that the virus they carried was *Zaire Ebola virus*. However, of several organs tested, only liver and spleen gave positive PCR results and the scientists could not actually isolate live virus from any of the animals. This suggests an extremely low level of infection in the virus-carrying bats. Also, none of the antibody-positive bats had detectable virus RNA, and conversely none of the virus RNA-positive bats had detectable antibodies. The scientists interpreted this intriguing finding as indicating that the RNA-positive bats were experiencing a primary Ebola infection and that once they had developed antibodies the virus was eliminated from their bodies. If true this means that Ebola causes a mild or silent acute infection in these bat species and persists in a colony by circulating continuously among its members.[18]

The three fruit bat species identified as potential reservoirs of Ebola, *Hysignathus monstrosus*, *Epomops franqueti*, and *Myoncteris torquata*, all fly long distances, with a range covering the five countries in central Africa where historically Ebola outbreaks have occurred. And since these possible reservoirs of Ebola were identified, antibodies to Ebola have been detected at low levels in other species of fruit bats.[19] One positive animal was found in Accra, Ghana belonging to the species *Eidolon helvum*. This is a migratory fruit bat that is common across the whole of Sub Saharan Africa, forming large roosts of several million animals, often in or near cities. When scientists radio-tagged the one Ebola antibody-positive animal from Accra they not only recorded its survival for over a year, indicating that Ebola infection had no ill effects on its health, but also tracked its migratory path of over 2,500km in that time period alone.[20]

Despite all the hype about fruit bats as the reservoir for Ebola, there is still a question mark over the validity of this assumption as no infectious virus has yet been isolated from any of the bat species implicated. Also, exactly how the virus jumps from bats to humans and non-human primates is not understood. Bats are commonly hunted and eaten as bush meat in central and west central Africa, giving a clear route of virus transmission through blood contact while catching, handling, and cooking infected bats. However, once cooked, eating an infected bat should not pose a threat as the heat required for cooking would inactivate the virus. Additionally, infection may occur through eating fruits contaminated with bat saliva. This is certainly supported by sightings of chimps and gorillas eating fruit from the same trees as fruit bats, particularly in the dry season when fruit is scarce.[21] Apparently fruit bats have a habit of test-biting fruit and then spitting it out, scattering chewed fruit spats under the trees in which they feed.[22] Clearly, if bat saliva contains Ebola virus then contaminated spats would be an obvious source of infection for other fruit-eating animals.

Recent detailed mapping studies to estimate the geographical area at risk of Ebola have included information on the bats' range and suspected distribution of their roosts as well as data on environmental factors such as vegetation, elevation, and temperature. If bats truly are the reservoir of Ebola then this has defined a much wider risk of Ebola infection in humans than was previously thought. Scientists now predict that certain areas in twenty-two separate countries across central and west Africa, inhabited by

22 million people, are at risk of Ebola.[23] They also stress that rapidly growing populations in Africa, for example in DRC where the population was around 20 million in 1976 and is now approximately 80 million, along with vastly increased availability of international air travel, indicate that much larger and more widespread epidemics could occur in future—a prediction which came true in 2014.

4

Ebola Strikes West Africa

The Catastrophic Events of 2014

In August 2014, WHO Secretary General Margaret Chan declared a 'Public Health Emergency of International Concern' in West Africa. For many people around the world this was the first indication that anything was amiss in West Africa, but by this time Ebola had already infected 2,274 people and killed 961 of them. An Ebola epidemic was spreading and Chan's announcement was admitting that it was out of control. Never before had an Ebola outbreak spread internationally or raged for so long.

Key events in the unfolding epidemic are shown in the timeline. Then finally, after six months of fighting a losing battle, it was obvious that an Ebola epidemic of unprecedented scale was raging in Guinea, Sierra Leone, and Liberia and that international help on the ground was essential to win the war against Ebola.

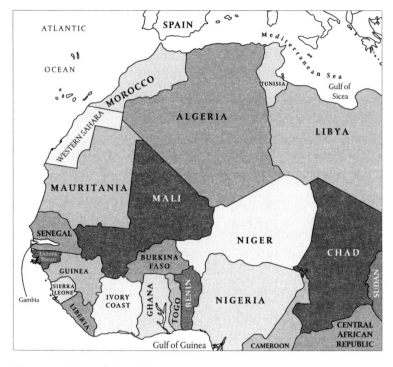

Figure 5 Map of West Africa.

2014 Ebola Epidemic Timeline
THE FIRST SIX MONTHS
See figures 5, 6, and 7.

MARCH 2014
>   **Guinea**—A mysterious, fatal disease strikes in the prefectures of Guéckédou and Macenta

MARCH
10th   **Guinea**—Local public health officials in Guéckédou alert the Ministry of Health

12th   **Guinea**—Local health officials inform MSF workers in Guéckédou

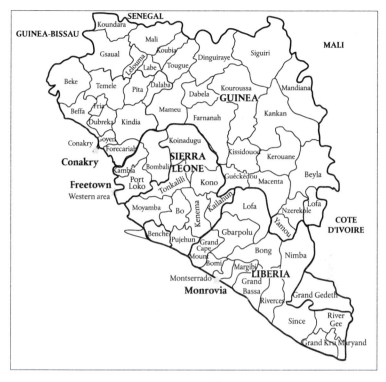

Figure 6   Maps of Guinea, Sierra Leone, and Liberia showing regions.

14th   **Guinea**—A team of experts from the Ministry of Health visit Guéckédou

18th   **Guinea**—MSF reinforcements arrive from Europe

22nd   **Guinea**—The mystery disease is diagnosed as Ebola

24th   **Guinea**—MSF build the first Ebola isolation centre in Guéckédou

31st   **Liberia**—Ebola cases diagnosed in Lofa and Nimba counties

By the end of March WHO reports a total of 112 Ebola cases with 70 deaths (Figure 7)

APRIL

1st   **Guinea**—Five experts from CDC arrive to assist the Guinean Ministry of Health and WHO Africa team in response to the Ebola outbreak

By the end of April WHO reports a total of 239 Ebola cases with 160 deaths

MAY

7th   **Guinea**—CDC team return to US satisfied that the Ebola outbreak is responding to control measures

12th   **Guinea**—Ebola reaches the capital, Conakry

26th   **Sierra Leone**—Ebola cases and deaths confirmed in Kailahun District

By the end of May WHO reports a total of 383 Ebola cases with 211 deaths

MAY

11th   **Sierra Leone**—Closes borders with Guinea and Liberia and shuts schools and cinemas in Ebola-affected areas

JUNE

15th   **Sierra Leone**—Ebola spreads to four further Districts

17th   **Liberia**—Ebola reaches the capital, Monrovia

21st   **Guinea, Sierra Leone, Liberia**—MSF declares the Ebola outbreak 'totally out of control' and calls for immediate, massive resources to stem virus spread

By the end of June WHO reports a total of 779 Ebola cases with 481 deaths

JULY

25th   **Sierra Leone**—Ebola reaches the capital, Freetown

25th   **Nigeria**—The first Ebola case confirmed in Lagos

27th   Liberia—International borders are closed and screening is introduced at the international airport. Schools and universities are closed, football matches banned, and the worst affected areas quarantined

27th   **Sierra Leone and Liberia**—The military used to enforce quarantine restrictions

By the end of July WHO report a total of 1,603 Ebola cases with 887 deaths

AUGUST

5th   **Guinea, Sierra Leone, and Liberia**—Major international airlines cancel flights to the capital cities

8th   **WHO** declares a Public Health Emergency of International Concern in West Africa

19th   Liberia—Angry youths storm a Quarantine Centre in West Point Township, Monrovia

20th   Liberia—President Sirleaf places a quarantine order on West Point and barricades the whole area

28th   **WHO** publish a plan for coordinating the international response to Ebola in West Africa. Many say 'too little too late'

29th   **Senegal**—The first Ebola case confirmed

30th   Liberia—The barricades around West Point removed; the Government admit they were a mistake

By the end of August WHO report a total of 3,707 Ebola cases with 1,808 deaths, but admit that these figures vastly underestimate the scale of the epidemic

SEPTEMBER

2nd   **MSF**—Workers on the ground warn the United Nations (UN) that the world is losing the battle against Ebola

18th   **UN** establishes a UN Mission for Ebola Emergency Response, the first ever created for a medical emergency

28th   **WHO** say 'The Ebola epidemic ravaging parts of West Africa is the most severe acute public health emergency seen in modern times. Never before in recorded history has a bio-safety level four pathogen infected so many people so quickly, over such a broad geographical area for so long.'

By the end of September WHO report a total of 7,492 cases with 3,439 deaths

*   *   *

Guinea, Sierra Leone, and Liberia sit side by side on the Atlantic coast of Africa. With a total population around 21.5 million, they each have a border with the other two while Guinea also borders Guinea Bissau, Senegal, and Mali, and both Guinea and Liberia border Côte d'Ivoire (Figure 5). Guinea, about the size of the UK and the largest and most populous of the three countries, forms a crescent of land around the northeast regions of Sierra Leone and Liberia. These three countries are presently among the poorest of developing countries, with GDPs ranking close to the lowest in the world. Health care facilities are inadequate, life expectancy is low (56–58 years), average fertility rates are high (around six births per adult female) as is infant mortality (up to 90 per 1,000 live births, compared to four to five per 1,000 in the Western world). Malnutrition and infectious diseases such as respiratory infections, malaria, and dysentery are rife. A combination of poverty, political unrest, corruption, human rights issues, high illiteracy, and poor infrastructure has also discouraged international trade and thereby prevented the population as a whole from benefiting from their countries' rich natural resources. All three countries are heavily dependent on international aid.

This sad state of affairs has its origins in the history of the region, with each country still emerging from decades of civil unrest. Following independence from their ruling powers the

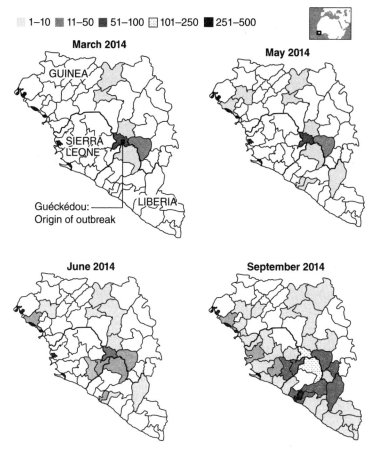

Figure 7   West Africa Ebola maps March 2014 to September 2014.

three countries experienced turbulent times, erupting into civil war in Sierra Leone and Liberia. Guinea avoided outright civil war and so became the main haven for refugees, with some two million arriving from Sierra Leone in the early 1990s and similar numbers from Liberia during its two civil wars in 1989–96 and 1999–2003. However, in the past decade all three countries have had elections, selecting presidents who are committed to ridding their countries of corruption. In 2014 an Ebola epidemic was the last thing that these emerging democracies could cope with.

* * *

We shall see how, when, and where the Guinean Ebola outbreak actually began in Chapter 7, but by the time it was recognized in March 2014 immediate, massive action was required to implement WHO guidelines for dealing with an Ebola outbreak which were formulated after the Kikwit outbreak in 1995. However, in a region that had never experienced Ebola before, there was no knowledge of how to act and no preparations for such an event had been made. So governments were starting from scratch and urgently needed protective clothing and training for health care workers, isolation centres for Ebola cases, personnel to trace and quarantine their contacts, community education and mobilization, and supervised safe and dignified burials.

The borders between Guinea, Sierra Leone, and Liberia, as well as those between Côte d'Ivoire and Guinea and Liberia, run through remote forested areas, are uncontrolled, and extremely porous. In addition, there are relatively easy road connections between these rural areas and densely populated cities, and recent upgrading of road networks in West Africa has greatly improved transport systems and thereby encouraged mobility. Masses of people routinely travel in 'route taxis'—minibuses designed to carry fifteen people but regularly plying the highways with up to twenty-five passengers along with their fruit and vegetables for market, their luggage, and occasional livestock as well. This, combined with leaky borders meant that more people were travelling more frequently and over longer distances than ever before. So once the virus had infiltrated rural villages it could easily find its way to all three capital cities. And this was exactly what happened.

The control measures implemented by governments were haphazard, inadequate, and ineffectual, and so the virus spread uncontrollably. With little coordination in response between the three countries, the virus moved freely throughout the region and numbers of new cases increased exponentially. WHO officials in Africa, whose role was to help and advise governments on just such an emergency, continued to believe that this outbreak would respond to implementation of the WHO guidelines that had served so well in the past. But the already fragile health services were simply overwhelmed by the scale of the problem, and all attempts to halt the spread of the virus failed.

When it became obvious that they were fighting a losing battle, government officials in Guinea began a cover-up. For the sake of maintaining international business links they purposely underplayed the number of Ebola cases and deaths, assuring the world that all was under control. Despite MSF's insistence that international help was needed, vital decisions were delayed and in consequence the early window of opportunity closed and thousands fell victim to Ebola.

One of the key factors that helped Ebola to get a firm grip in the region was the population's deep mistrust of governments, engendered by the years of turmoil in West Africa. So when a new and mysterious disease struck, conspiracy theories abounded. The population had never seen or heard of Ebola, and now many doubted the explanation of their governments for the sudden, lethal plague. What was urgently needed at this moment was an authoritative figure like Jean-Jacques Muyembe-Tamfum in Kikwit, DRC, who explained Ebola in terms that local people could understand. But no such 'local hero' existed, and at that time, Muyembe was busy controlling another Ebola outbreak in

Buende district, DRC. So people preferred to believe that the disease was caused by evil spirits or was a punishment by god because they had 'lost their way'; beliefs compounded by certain religious leaders. The Catholic Archbishop of Liberia reportedly preached that 'one of the major transgressions against god, for which he may be punishing Liberia, is the act of homosexuality'[1] while others convinced their followers that good Christians and believers were safe from Ebola, using texts from the Bible to support their claim: 'For nations shall rise against nations, and kingdom against kingdom: and there shall be famines, and pestilences, and earthquakes, in divers places. All these are the beginning of sorrows…But he that shall endure unto the end, the same shall be saved.'[2]

Many blamed the governments themselves for deaths of their relatives and friends, and were sceptical about the presence of foreign doctors and their Western medicine. In Sierra Leone, some even thought that Ebola was engineered by the West to control their population growth and gain economic influence over the country.[3] With all these misguided rumours and theories circulating, the sick and their families naturally turned to the traditional healers they knew and trusted rather than taking their loved ones to foreign doctors in the hastily constructed quarantine and treatment centres, which they regarded as death traps.

Inevitably, as the death toll climbed, tensions rose and occasionally erupted into violence. This is exactly what happened in West Point, one of Monrovia's most densely packed slums. With around 75,000 people packed into 2.5 km² (1 square mile) West Point has no running water and just four public toilets. Ebola reached the township in August 2014, and in no time the one small clinic was overflowing with dead and dying Ebola victims. A disused school was hastily commandeered as a quarantine centre, but with no doctors or nurses, and no separation between suspected and confirmed cases, those who did not have Ebola were very likely to catch it there. Unsurprisingly, when it was rumoured that Ebola sufferers from around the city were being imported into West Point quarantine centre, tempers flared. Just four days after it opened, a gang of youths stormed the centre, releasing its inmates and dragging their contaminated mattresses into the streets.

Officials panicked, fearing that left to their own devices the West Point rioters would disseminate Ebola throughout the capital city. President Sirleaf ordered the quarantining of the whole township for twenty-one days—the incubation period of Ebola. Overnight barricades went up, patrolled by armed guards. A nightly curfew was imposed and ships guarded the port, cutting off all escape routes by sea. No one could enter or leave the area; West Point residents were trapped. Riots ensued and when troops retaliated with gun fire and tear gas a 15-year-old boy was fatally wounded. Seventeen days later the government admitted the folly of their hasty action and the barricades came down. They had alienated the inhabitants of West Point and achieved nothing in return.

* * *

In rural areas of West Africa there are deeply ingrained traditional beliefs and secret societies are particularly active, forming strong and powerful social networks. These non-political, non-religious societies control all local behaviours, including burial rites. Here, as in DRC, death is often regarded as *the* most important life event and passing to the afterlife is only achieved by meticulous performance of burial rituals by friends and family of the deceased. And if safe passage does not occur then the dead will stay to haunt the living. A funeral is also a celebration attended by as many friends and relations as possible. Until recently that would have been only those who heard the news by word of mouth, but now that virtually everyone owns a mobile phone, huge numbers of people can be notified within minutes and funerals have become large, social gatherings, sometimes lasting for several days. As in previous Ebola outbreaks, these funerals posed a major risk for Ebola spread.

At the start of the epidemic in Guinea efforts were made to block this route of virus transmission by raising awareness about Ebola virus, the disease, and the hazards of traditional burials. Health care workers and officials visited villages to discuss alterations to traditional funeral practices, but many villagers were suspicious of these outsiders, fearing that their cultural traditions were being threatened. Indeed, some zealous heads of secret societies undermined the delicate work of those promoting safe burials by persuading villagers not to change their ways but to adhere to traditional burial rituals. On one terrible occasion in September 2014, a team of health care workers, local officials, and journalists visited the village of Wome in Southern Guinea to discuss the outbreak and its consequences. Violence broke out,[4] and although no one knows exactly what happened, from the eight bodies later recovered it was clear that the team had been attacked with rocks, clubs, and machetes. Six villagers were later arrested while the rest fled.

Before international help arrived, hospitals in Guinea, Sierra Leone, and Liberia were overflowing with Ebola victims, and staff were struggling to cope. At this stage the large government hospital in Kenema, a city in Sierra Leone near the origin of the outbreak in Guinea, was designated as a major Ebola treatment centre. Before the epidemic hit, the hospital had been a centre for Lassa fever treatment, but it was soon overwhelmed with Ebola cases. Staff lacked any expertise in caring for Ebola patients and had little in the way of personal protective equipment. Many health care workers at the hospital caught Ebola, and prominent among them was Sheik Hummarr Khan, lead physician at the hospital and well known and loved in the local community. He headed up the fight against Ebola in Kenema until July 2014 when he succumbed to the disease.[5] His death triggered rumours in the town suggesting that Ebola was a myth invented by nurses who were killing people in the hospital and even performing cannibalistic rituals on their bodies. Riots broke out, and although these were quickly quelled by police using tear gas, the whole incident left the community with a lack of trust in hospitals and Western medicine. Clearly they urgently needed to see some positive results in the form of cured Ebola sufferers returning to their families rather than bodies being sent home for burial. But this would only happen when more, better-equipped treatment centres with fully trained staff were up and running.

*   *   *

While the Ebola epidemic was raging in Guinea, Sierra Leone, and Liberia through the summer and autumn of 2014, WHO's worst fears were realized—further international spread. Travellers carried Ebola to Nigeria, Senegal, and Mali while repatriation of Western volunteers with Ebola resulted in onward spread in Spain and the US.

In Nigeria the index case was 40-year-old Patrick Sawyer, a Liberian civil servant from the Ministry of Finance, who jetted into Nigeria carrying the virus with him. His journey began in Monrovia on July 20, 2014, when he was clearly already suffering symptoms of Ebola. But as temperature screening was not implemented at the airport until the following week, he boarded a plane bound for Murtata Muhammed International airport, Lagos, unhindered. He vomited on the plane, again on arrival in Lagos—Africa's busiest airport—and once again in the private car that took him to the First Consultant Hospital in Lagos. When questioned, Sawyer denied contact with any Ebola sufferers, although it later transpired that his sister had recently died of the disease in Liberia. Not only had he visited her in hospital but he had also attended her funeral and traditional burial ceremony. At the First Consultant Hospital Sawyer insisted he was suffering an attack of malaria, but, against his will, he was detained for blood tests. These proved that he was suffering from Ebola from which he died five days later.

Because of the provisional diagnosis of malaria, the health workers caring for Sawyer initially wore no protective clothing. Nine later developed Ebola, four of whom died. Amongst them was Dr Ameyo Stella Adadevoh, who, despite Sawyer's protestations, alerted local health officials to the possibility of an Ebola case and insisted on isolating him until the diagnosis was confirmed. But Sawyer was equally determined to get to the conference he had travelled to Lagos to attend, and called government colleagues to assist him. They then accused Adadevoh of kidnapping him! When Sawyer became aggressive and removed his intravenous line, thereby contaminating the whole room with his virus-laden blood, Adadevoh physically restrained him. It is no wonder that she contracted the deadly virus from which she died.[6]

Adadevoh's selfless act was mirrored by many across West Africa where close to 900 Ebola experts, doctors, nurses, and carers caught Ebola and over 500 died from the disease they were so bravely fighting.

Lagos, Africa's largest city, has 21 million inhabitants and some of Africa's worst slums. Government health officials, describing the city as 'a powder keg' in relation to Ebola, knew that if the virus got loose in Lagos it would cause a raging epidemic with an enormous death toll and almost certain global spread. To his credit, President Buhari offered unlimited funds to control the outbreak, and Nigerian health officials, aided by experts from WHO and CDC, took immediate action. They traced all of Sawyer's 898 contacts and isolated them until the danger period was over. Unfortunately, one contact, an official who accompanied Sawyer in the car from Lagos airport to First Consultant Hospital, managed to slip through the net. He fled quarantine and travelled 600km to Port Harcourt, the oil capital of Nigeria with over a million citizens. There he holed up in a hotel, receiving treatment from a private doctor, Ike Enemuo. Although he survived Ebola, the virus jumped to Enemuo, who continued to see, and operate on, patients until he fell ill on August 11. He died in hospital on August 22 where his illness was retrospectively diagnosed as Ebola on August 27. During the critical infectious period Enemuo accumulated over 200 contacts, sixty of whom were regarded as high risk. Virtually all were traced and quarantined for twenty-one days. Remarkably, only three developed Ebola—Enemuo's wife and a doctor and a patient from the hospital. Overall Nigeria had twenty Ebola cases and eight deaths. The country was declared Ebola free on October

20, 2014—a triumph for Nigeria and a great relief for the whole world.

It was those travelling by road who carried the virus across the border from Guinea to Senegal and Mali. Fortunately though, as neighbours to the most severely affected countries, both Senegal and Mali were prepared for this event and virus spread was minimal. Ebola reached Senegal in August 2014, when an infected Guinean man arrived in the capital, Dakar. Health officials traced and quarantined seventy-four of his contacts but none developed Ebola. Mali received two influxes of Ebola in 2014, the first carried by a 2-year-old girl who travelled by bus from Guinea with her grandmother after her mother died of Ebola. The child was already unwell when they set out on the journey and on arrival Ebola was confirmed. She died three days later. Over 100 of her contacts were traced and monitored but none contracted Ebola. Ebola entered Mali for a second time in November 2014 when a Guinean Imam visited the capital, Bamako. He was treated at the Pasteur Clinic in Bamako, where he died before the diagnosis of Ebola was made. This spawned a small cluster of Ebola cases including a nurse at the clinic who died of the disease. Over 256 of their contacts were traced and quarantined but the virus spread no further. Overall Mali had eight Ebola cases and six deaths. The country was declared Ebola free on January 18, 2015.

For many in the West the first uncomfortable recognition that Ebola could strike close to home came in August 2014 when the repatriation of two American missionaries who contracted Ebola in Liberia hit the headlines. Over the following months there was a constant trickle of foreign volunteers being repatriated to the US and Europe, around twenty-four in all, of whom five died. In Spain a Catholic priest evacuated from Liberia in October died in the

Hospital Carlos III in Madrid. Despite precautions, the virus jumped to a nurse who had cared for him; the first confirmed Ebola case to contract the disease outside Africa. She survived and none of her fifty contacts developed the disease. Similarly, in the US, where eleven Ebola cases were treated, the virus jumped to two nurses in the Texas Health Presbyterian Hospital in Dallas. Both survived and the virus spread no further. But these cases caused intense media interest and a panicky and hysterical over-reaction by the authorities. With no privacy afforded to the patients, and updates on their progress broadcast hourly, news of the sufferers of a life-threatening illness was beamed around the globe. In the US, West African residents experienced discrimination and alienation while volunteers returning from West Africa were threatened with quarantine. In Spain officials even euthanized the dog belonging to an Ebola victim in case it was the source of her infection! Clearly those responsible for these actions had no understanding of how Ebola spreads. As Charles M Blow wrote in the *New York Times*: 'On Ebola, the possible has overtaken the probable, gobbling it up in a high-anxiety, low-information frenzy of frayed nerves...We aren't battling a virus in this country as much as a mania, one whipped up by reactionary politicians and irresponsible media. We should be following the science in responding to the threat, but instead we are being led by silliness.'[7]

* * *

The stark contrast between the successful Ebola response in Nigeria, Senegal, and Mali and the uncontrolled spread of the epidemic in Guinea, Sierra Leone, and Liberia was down to these countries being well prepared for the event. Their governments, with fair warning of the threat from neighbouring countries, reacted quickly and efficiently to prevent uncontrolled virus spread. On each occasion the index case was rapidly identified and contacts swiftly traced and monitored. But, as discussed in Chapter 7, it was quite a different story in Guinea in March 2014 when it took some very clever detective work to uncover the index case for the whole epidemic.

5

~~~

Ebola Epidemic

The Fight Back

By September 2014 the doubling times for the epidemic were sixteen days in Guinea, thirty days in Sierra Leone, and twenty-three days in Liberia. Based on these values, WHO made the grim prediction that 'the number of cases and of deaths from EVD [Ebola virus disease] are expected to continue increasing from hundreds to thousands per week in the coming months' and that, assuming no change in control measures, the cumulative numbers of confirmed and probable cases would exceed 20,000 in total by the beginning of November 2014.[1] Fortunately, WHO had slightly overestimated perhaps because by now their plans for Ebola control were being implemented and international help was at hand.

* * *

The WHO Ebola Response Roadmap was published on August 28, 2014, by which time there had been over 3,000 Ebola cases and 1,400 deaths in Guinea, Sierra Leone, and Liberia, close to 40% of which had occurred in the previous three weeks.[2] This Roadmap represented a framework for controlling the epidemic in the three worst affected countries whilst also rapidly managing any international spread. The response was divided into three clear phases:

Phase 1—to reverse the rising trend in new Ebola cases within three months by providing a 'massively scaled and coordinated international response...to support affected and at-risk countries'

Phase 2—to stop ongoing Ebola transmission worldwide within six to nine months

Phase 3—to achieve and sustain a resilient zero for Ebola cases

While the response was designed to assist governments and NGOs in controlling the epidemic, the UN provided a further plan for underpinning the response by ensuring vital supplies such as food, water, sanitation, health care, and education during the response and longer term recovery phase. In addition, WHO, together with the World Bank, would coordinate financial support (with appeals to domestic and international governments, development banks, and private-sector financing) and provide resource-tracking for the Roadmap.

The plan outlined by WHO was based on strategies that had been tried and tested in Ebola outbreaks described in earlier chapters; rapid diagnosis, treatment in isolation centres, case contact tracing and monitoring, safe burials, and full community engagement in the overall plan. However, WHO acknowledged that the unique feature of *this* epidemic was intense Ebola spread among urban populations, where the virus moved so fast that at any one time the actual number of new cases was probably around four times the reported figure. In towns and cities, where hospitals were generally overflowing with cases, new methods were required to control Ebola spread. WHO planned to develop complementary approaches with local inhabitants forming their own teams of community-based care workers and dedicated burial teams to provide safe and dignified funerals. Household case contacts would be isolated either in their own homes or in community isolation centres, and banned from non-essential movement in and out of containment areas. All cases and contacts would be prohibited from travelling and exit screening at international airports, seaports, and land border crossings would be implemented. All mass gatherings, including schools, markets, and sports events, but excluding religious services and Ebola training sessions, were banned until the intensity of transmission reduced.

By now, over 240 Ebola cases and 120 deaths had occurred among health care workers, giving them around a 25-times higher risk of infection than the general adult population. Thus WHO stressed education and training for *everyone* involved in the fight against Ebola, and provision of adequate quantities of personal protection equipment for them all. In September WHO began training nurses and other health care workers in infection control and the use of personal protection equipment to prepare them for work in hospitals and the new Ebola treatment centres that were being constructed. The need for these sessions escalated as numbers of volunteers rapidly increased, and in Sierra Leone they eventually took over several rooms at the National Stadium in Freetown, empty because of the ban on sports events. With an emphasis on social mobilization throughout the training, organizers hoped that trainees would become 'mouthpieces' in their communities to help quell the flow of misguided rumours.

*   *   *

Several studies indicated that most Ebola transmission was occurring in the community. Indeed, a survey following chains of infection in Conakry, Guinea, showed that in March 2014, before implementation of infection control measures, 35% of infections occurred in hospitals, 15% at funerals, and the remaining 50% arose in the community. However, by the end of April, when control measures were in place, these figures had changed to 9%, 4%, and 82% respectively, with 72% of community transmissions being within the family.[3] Clearly, transmission in hospitals and at funerals was coming under control by strict adherence to infection control procedures by hospital staff and dedicated burial teams. But this was certainly not the case for transmission within the community.

The reasons for the dramatic number of community infections in this epidemic were twofold. On one hand, for all the reasons outlined earlier, families often preferred to nurse their loved ones at home rather than moving them to a hospital from which they were unlikely to return. On the other hand, there was a huge lack of available beds in hospitals and health care centres and often no means of transporting the sick to them. In November, the average time between developing Ebola symptoms (and therefore becoming infectious) and being admitted to an isolation unit in Sierra Leone was four days, with some cases waiting more than a week.[4] Indeed, there were stories of very sick patients dying in taxis outside hospitals while waiting for someone inside to die and vacate a bed. As a result, patients at the late, and most infectious, stage of Ebola disease remained in the community as a potent source of infection.

The mission for the immediate phase 1 of the response was to rapidly build the infrastructure for isolating 70% of new infections and ensure that 70% of burials were safe. If this could be achieved then WHO predicted that by the beginning of December

2014 the case reproductive number, R_0, would drop below one, showing that numbers of new cases were beginning to fall. Implementation of the WHO Roadmap phase 1 got UNDER WAY in earnest in autumn 2014.

*   *   *

Although Guinea, Sierra Leone, and Liberia are neighbours, they have very different histories and affiliations. While Guinea, formally known as French Guinea, was colonized by the French in the 1890s and is French speaking, Sierra Leone and Liberia are English-speaking countries that were created as havens for freed slaves towards the end of the slave trade era by British (in 1787) and by US (in 1821) philanthropists respectively. With this background in mind, France took the lead on Ebola control in Guinea, the UK in Sierra Leone, and the US in Liberia, each aiding the respective government by providing technical, financial, and logistical support. In general the epidemic was said to be mainly rural in Guinea, urban in Liberia, and both rural and urban in Sierra Leone—the worst affected country at the time. However, all three countries were suffering similar overwhelming logistical and social problems for which the overarching solution was the same. The following is an account of the fight back in Sierra Leone.

When the UK joined the fight against Ebola on the ground in Sierra Leone there were around 500 new cases every week in the country, and, with the value of R_0 as high as 2.5 in the worst affected areas, the battle was to get this figure to below one as quickly as possible. As a result of its turbulent history, Sierra Leone completely lacked the infrastructure to manage an epidemic of this size and ferocity. Even the emergency call service had to be set up from scratch, an emergency number (117) created and made public, and a call centre established. The new National

Ebola Response Centre, the command and control centre for the whole Ebola response in Sierra Leone, was headed by Palo Conteh, Sierra Leonean ex-Minister of Defence. This huge enterprise, which took over the court buildings in Freetown, worked closely with the government and international agencies to provide the backbone of the response—infrastructure, commodities, training, and management, all on a massive scale. Meanwhile, at the British Council Offices in Freetown, Lieutenant Colonel Andy Garrow, a Royal Engineer, was heading up Ebola Command and Control for Freetown. With a staff of 1,600, he was responsible for coordinating the management of Ebola victims in the city; everything from dispatching ambulances, blood collection and transportation, Ebola testing of the living and the dead, contact tracing, quarantining, and safe burials. In what must qualify as the understatement of the year, referring to his complex job Garrow remarked: 'there are a lot of moving parts, and everything needs to be coordinated'.[5]

Mathematical models used to test out various options for controlling the epidemic indicated that R_0 would eventually fall below one if the time interval between a patient becoming symptomatic and being admitted to an isolation unit was cut by just one to two days.[6] So the aim of the UK strategic plan was to isolate at least 70% of Ebola cases within three days of their symptoms developing. The ideal way to achieve this was to ramp up the programme for actively seeking early Ebola cases in the community and chasing their contacts followed by rapidly isolating the former in fully staffed and equipped hospitals and monitoring the latter. But with up to ten trained staff required to monitor the contacts of just one case, this was deemed impossible with the manpower available. Also, as hospitals were already overrun with Ebola cases, isolation of even more cases from the community could not be achieved until phase 1 of the response had dramatically increased the available bed capacity. To cope with this dilemma a two-pronged strategy was devised: (1) self-referral of possible Ebola sufferers (known as 'passive case finding') with isolation in community care centres, and (2) provision of more, better-staffed and equipped treatment centres.

The idea of community care centres was to provide small, local isolation centres for case contacts and suspected Ebola cases with quick referral to hospital if/when Ebola diagnosis was confirmed.[7] Estimates suggested that around 200 of these would be required in Sierra Leone and in practical terms this meant rapidly building pop-up community units in Ebola affected areas—often just three to five beds in a tent or an existing building adapted for the purpose—where suspected cases could receive basic health care and would avoid infecting their family members. Admission to the centres would be voluntary and although the issue of using incentives to persuade those suspected of incubating Ebola to self-refer to a care centre was discussed during the planning process, it was left open at the time and in reality was not required. In many communities there was a deep-rooted fear of Ebola sufferers and Ebola survivors, with stigmatization of survivors and their families. So an important facet of this plan was engagement with the local community and religious leaders to develop understanding, acceptance, and ownership of the overall plan, particularly the concept of isolation of Ebola sufferers outside their homes to prevent the disease spreading. Therefore, wherever possible, carers for the centres were volunteers who lived in, and were trusted by, the local community who had been given basic training and supplied with protective clothing.

Nevertheless, using community care centres was a step into the unknown. Most people with Ebola-like symptoms would turn out not to have Ebola but more common diseases like gastroenteritis, pneumonia, and malaria. So the danger was that these Ebola-negative individuals would actually catch Ebola while being assessed in a centre. As there was no time to test the advantages and disadvantages of community care centres on the ground, the best alternative was to model the system mathematically and weigh the benefits against the risks. This study showed that 'CCCs [community care centres] could reduce the number of Ebola virus disease cases in the community if 1) the probability of Ebola-virus negative patients being exposed to the virus is low and 2) there is reduction in virus transmission as a result of infected patients being in CCC.' But that 'the CCC approach is little tested in the field and could be harmful if infection control in CCCs is worse than in the community or if Ebola virus-negative patients have a high risk of exposure to virus'.[8]

With this result, the decision was taken to proceed, accepting that extreme care had to be taken to prevent *amplifying* Ebola in community care centres rather than controlling its spread. The whole plan needed sensitive handling in each community and teams of social workers were employed alongside carers and medical personnel to explain the plan in terms that could be understood by people with no previous experience of the disease or comprehension of contagion via a kiss or a handshake. Strongly held religious beliefs as well as the stigma of having suffered, or having a family member who suffered, from Ebola could upset the plan by driving some to hide Ebola cases and perform secret traditional burials.

* * *

In October WHO calculated that there were just 326 hospital beds for Ebola sufferers in Sierra Leone, but by November six new treatment centres were under construction, providing a further 880 beds when completed. Funded by the UK Government and built by local contractors working alongside British Army Royal Engineers, the first of these centres opened in Kerry Town, 30km west of Freetown, on November 5, 2014. The facility had the capacity to treat up to eighty Ebola patients with an additional twenty beds in a specialist unit for health care workers, and was managed by Save the Children and staffed by 200 volunteers. Yet, from the start it was obvious that this treatment centre was not ideally situated. Kerry Town itself is neither a large town nor a transport hub where Ebola might be expected to flourish. In fact it is so small that it does not even feature on most maps of the country. So why was a treatment centre built there? Because, even in this dire emergency, the 'not in my back yard' mentality was still a powerful force, and so it was the best site available at the time. As a result, the sick and dying had to be transported further from their homes, blood samples from suspected cases in hospitals and care centres took longer to reach the laboratory, and returning bodies to their village for burial became a time-consuming task.

Completion of Kerry Town Ebola Treatment Centre was followed by centres of similar size in Makeni and Port Loko in Sierra Leone Northern Province, Moyamba in the Southern Province, Hastings, 24km east of Freetown, and Goderich in a western suburb of Freetown (Figure 8). All were up and running by the end of December 2014, and functioned alongside several additional treatment centres constructed and run by other foreign governments and NGOs.

Each treatment centre was carefully designed with separate high- (red) and low- (green) risk zones. In the high-risk zone staff wore complete personal protective clothing at all times—goggles,

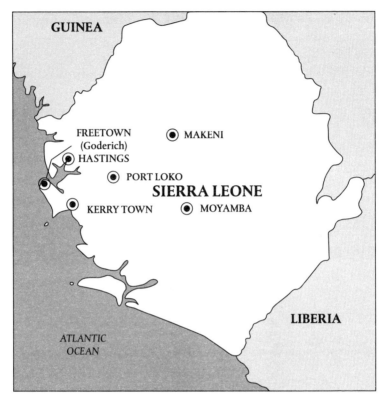

Figure 8 Map of Sierra Leone showing location of UK Ebola Treatment Centres.

mask, impervious yellow plastic suit, plastic apron with their name on the front so that fellow staff and patients could recognize them, chemical-resistant gloves and rubber boots (Figure 9). Staff always worked in pairs—the buddy system—helping their partners into and out of the cumbersome 'uniform' and checking each other to ensure that once inside no area of skin was exposed. Because of the tropical climate, full personal protective equipment could only be worn for about forty minutes at a stretch before it became unbearably hot and sweaty inside. And when,

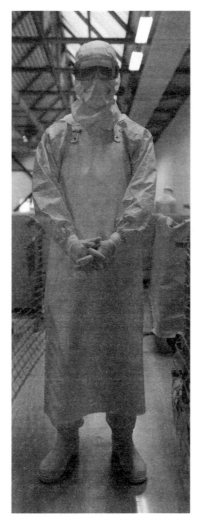

Figure 9   Personal protective equipment.

early in the epidemic, personal protective equipment was in short supply, thicker less flexible suits designed for the chemical industry had to be worn, so accentuating the discomfort. Staff going on duty in the high-risk zone first entered a briefing area where they met the changeover team and received instructions on their tasks before proceeding to the changing area to don their personal protection equipment.

With no specific treatment for Ebola, care duties mainly involved keeping patients as clean and comfortable as possible, encouraging them to drink or, where this was not possible, initiating intravenous rehydration. Bodies of the dead had to be rendered safe by disinfecting them and placing them in body bags in the high-risk zone before they could be released to the family for burial. The extremely lonely, disorientating experience of being confined to an isolation ward meant that carers needed to interact with patients as much as possible and, on occasion, supervise family visits.

With their duties over, staff left the high-risk zone by a separate route and removed their suits, again with the help of a buddy. Used suits and other non-recyclable material were burnt in an incinerator, often just a 'burn pit' within the high-risk zone, while the exiting staff disinfected themselves before re-entering the low-risk zone. This area contained all the support facilities—offices, pharmacy, stores, meeting areas, and the all-important laundry where recyclable items were washed, and boots scrubbed, in chlorinated water.

Kerry Town treatment centre was constructed from scratch on an area of bush and scrub. It comprised some prefabricated blocks, wards of canvas on concrete bases, and a huge generator in the centre of the low-risk zone (Figure 10). Patients with Ebola-like symptoms entered a high-risk zone through a reception/waiting area where they were assessed and triaged. Only those with symptoms that conformed to the WHO case definition of Ebola—fever plus three other symptoms from a list including fatigue, rash,

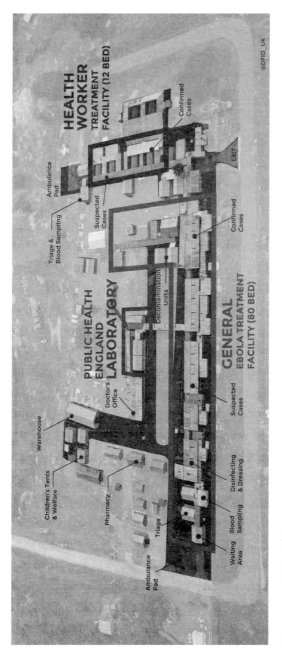

Figure 10 Map of Kerry Town treatment centre.

head and muscle aches, vomiting, diarrhoea, abdominal pain, and unexpected bleeding, were tested for Ebola and admitted to a holding ward to await the results. The centre had three holding wards designed to minimize Ebola spread inside the facility—one for low-likelihood cases with no contact history, one for high-risk wet cases (with diarrhoea and/or vomiting), and one for dry, high-likelihood cases. Wet cases were obviously the most infectious and so, to quote the lead doctor at Kerry Town, 'If you don't have Ebola then the most dangerous thing to have is gastroenteritis.' But he was quick to confirm that no virus transmission had occurred in the Kerry Town treatment centre wet holding ward. Once the test results were known, negative cases were discharged while positive cases were assigned to one of the three isolation wards depending on the type and severity of their symptoms, with a convalescent ward at the end of the line for those lucky enough to survive the disease.

*   *   *

Key to the success of the overall Ebola control plan in West Africa was rapid diagnosis of suspected cases. Then infected individuals reporting to community care or treatment centres could be rapidly isolated and contact tracing initiated while the uninfected could leave as soon as possible, so minimizing their risk of becoming infected whilst on the premises. Rapid PCR-based Ebola diagnostic kits had been on the market for some time by 2014 but handling potential Ebola virus-containing test samples required a containment level three facility with highly trained staff wearing personal protective equipment. Such a facility did not exist in West Africa in 2014. Early in the outbreak the European Union sent a mobile laboratory to Guéckédou, Guinea, for rapid Ebola testing on the assumption that this would be sufficient to cope

with the outbreak. But as cases increased this was far from adequate for all the tests required. During August and September
2014, South Africa, Canada, and China each opened mobile Ebola
testing laboratories in Sierra Leone, but again these were insufficient to cope with the growing epidemic, so that by November it
took five or more days to get a result—a period during which
cases remained in the community and their contacts dispersed.

In September 2014, Dr Tim Brooks, Head of the Rare and
Imported Pathogens Laboratory at Public Health England (PHE),
Porton Down, Salisbury, UK, was given the task of setting up a
country-wide Ebola testing service in Sierra Leone with a maximum turnaround time of twenty-four hours. Brooks' job at PHE
includes responding to any national or international emergency
that requires microbiological testing, so he jets off to wherever
laboratory facilities are needed in a hurry be it following a hurri-
cane or an earthquake, when cholera threatens, or, indeed, when
Ebola strikes West Africa. On this occasion, Brooks and his team
had just one month to plan before he headed for Sierra Leone in
October 2014 to set up a laboratory in Kerry Town alongside the
treatment centre then under construction. This was the first of
three laboratories that Brooks established. 'I have never worked so
hard in my life,' he says of the period between October 2014 and
the beginning of January 2015, during which he stayed at Kerry
Town but travelled around the country working against the clock
to get the new laboratories up and running. By November the
Kerry Town laboratory was ready to open and this was followed
by laboratories attached to the treatment centres at Makeni and
Port Loko.

The laboratories were staffed by British volunteers with expertise in virology who attended an intensive, five-day training course

at PHE before undertaking a five-week stint in Sierra Leone. For maximum safety, each new arrival worked alongside someone who had a few weeks' experience of the laboratory testing and safety protocols, and they worked in shifts so that laboratories could function daily from six in the morning until ten at night. Samples arrived in double, sealed bags which had been transported in chlorine solution. The gowned, masked, and double-gloved technicians placed the sample bags into a flexible film isolator where the tubes were removed from the bags, dunked in disinfectant, and then opened and the samples decontaminated. Only when chemical decontamination was complete were the samples safe to be removed from the cabinet and tested on the open bench. From then on it was a rapid, routine PCR test, each run taking around four hours to complete.

Professor Ian Goodfellow, Head of the Division of Virology at the University of Cambridge, UK, volunteered for a five-week stint in Sierra Leone in early November 2014 and was a team leader in the Makeni laboratory by the end of the month. When he arrived the laboratory was just a brick shell in the middle of a building site, so he spent the first week unloading lorries, opening boxes, setting up equipment, and improvising where essential pieces of kit were missing. So a sawn-off plastic ketchup bottle was combined with an empty cotton bud container to provide a receptacle for chlorine solution inside the isolator, and with no piped water, bottled water was used for everything from making up reagents to swabbing the floor until a bore hole was sunk on site. Goodfellow describes the working conditions in the laboratory, with eight hours a day inside hot and sweaty protective clothing and eyes streaming from the chlorine disinfectant, as 'quite challenging'. But the experience must have been a rewarding one because he returned to Sierra Leone for another five weeks in Makeni in February 2015.

* * *

The safety of volunteers, who were risking their lives to assist in the Ebola response, was paramount. All UK Ebola Response Team members in Sierra Leone were banned from travelling in taxis because these vehicles were used for transporting Ebola victims, either before or after death, and were often not reliably disinfected thereafter. Other restrictions varied according to the authority running each treatment centre; at Kerry Town, Save the Children officials insisted that staff be confined to the centre and their living quarters while volunteers at Makeni treatment centre, run by International Medical Corps, were free to wander around the town. But there was more to consider than just the threat of Ebola. In fact, strange as it may seem, even at the height of the epidemic it was deemed more likely that a volunteer would sustain a serious injury—usually in a road traffic accident—than catch Ebola. As the Sierra Leone Guide Book warns: 'Serious road accidents are quite frequent in Sierra Leone owing to the hazardous driving conditions, poor vehicle maintenance and erratic driving. All roads are un-lit and pot-holes are common, especially during the rainy season…The emergency service response to accidents in Freetown is very slow and unreliable. Outside the capital you should assume that there would be no emergency service response to an accident.'[9]

So, while the Royal Air Force flew any volunteers with sus-pected Ebola back to England for isolation and treatment at the Royal Free Hospital in London, a converted cargo ship, Royal Fleet Auxiliary Argus, containing a 100-bed hospital, an intensive care facility, and 300 staff, sailed to Sierra Leone and anchored off-shore ready to deal with volunteers suffering from any medical emergencies other than Ebola. In the event these facilities were not used to anything like their capacity, but, according to Brooks, the ship's helicopter was invaluable in ferrying equipment and personnel to and fro during the construction of treatment centres and laboratories.

*   *   *

By the end of December 2014, with several new treatment and community care centres in operation, phase 1 of the WHO Roadmap was complete and beginning to show results. Although numbers of Ebola cases and deaths were still rising week by week, the rise was noticeably slowing and the value of R_0 was edging closer to one. The total number of cases had now reached 20,206 with 7,904 reported deaths. Sierra Leone still experienced the most cases: 2,901 in November and 1,974 in December, with a total of 9,446 for the whole epidemic to date.

For Brooks the turning point came in January 2015 when he first witnessed a fall in the number of samples sent for Ebola testing. He also saw a drop in positive test results from around 50% to 10%. This was a good indication that Sierra Leone had turned the corner, and on January 28 WHO reported that, for the first time since June 2014, less than 100 cases had been reported that week (thirty in Guinea, sixty-five in Sierra Leone, and four in Liberia).[10] Everyone could see that the epidemic was waning, while also admitting that the road to complete virus elimination might be a long one.

*   *   *

The mission for phase 2 of the WHO Roadmap in West Africa was to enhance capacity for case finding, contact tracing, and community engagement. So in January 2015 it was time to increase surveillance activities by not only searching for case contacts but also going into communities to identify new cases and follow transmission chains by house-to-house searches (*active* as opposed to *passive* case finding). Key to the success of this labour-intensive plan was building bridges with local communities, many of which had been alienated by the perceived invasion of their traditional lifestyle due to the single-mindedness of phase 1 activities. Now it was essential to work *with* local community leaders and draw on their help as much as possible so that they took ownership of the overall plan. Community volunteers were needed to join burial teams and to carry out intensified surveillance, including the house-to-house searches for new and hidden cases. In particular, it was important to ask valued members of a community, such as nurses, midwives, and traditional healers, to join in, in order to lend credibility to the response effort.

On the whole phase 2 of the WHO Roadmap worked well. Once Ebola sufferers began returning, healed, to their families, rumours were dispelled and most communities engaged with the Ebola response and took responsibility for it. Inevitably there were pockets of resistance that kept the epidemic alive. In Guinea, for example, in May 2015, when a taxi full of passengers was stopped for a routine check a corpse was discovered sitting in the back, wearing T-shirt, jeans, and sunglasses. This turned out to be the body of a relative of the fellow passengers who had died of Ebola and was being transported home for burial. The six people riding with the body were arrested and placed in isolation in prison to await trial on a charge of violating the health emergency if they survived for twenty-one days' quarantine without dying of Ebola.

On the other side of the coin, there were encouraging stories demonstrating that outbreaks in close-knit communities could, with sensitive handling, result in community cooperation. Two such outbreaks occurred in the slums of Freetown. The first was in Aberdeen, a coastal township inhabited by fishermen and their families. Here around 10,000 people lived in makeshift shacks on or near the beach with no clean running water, no waste disposal, and no sewage system apart from four toilets built by Save the Children to serve the whole community. The beach area was piled high with rubbish and human excreta and was foraged by roaming packs of dogs. This was just the kind of overcrowded, unhygienic environment where Ebola thrived. The virus arrived in February 2015, brought to the community by fishermen returning from a trip at sea.

Small fishing craft often met up with similar boats from other villages along the coast, forming rafts of boats that remained at sea for several days. This contact between fishermen from along the coast introduced Ebola to Aberdeen, with over twenty cases occurring simultaneously in February 2015. Dr Katrina Roper, an epidemiologist from Melbourne, Australia, took part in the fight against the virus in Aberdeen, heading a WHO Ebola Response Team of epidemiologists and locally employed District Surveillance Officers. For several months they worked frantically, summoning ambulances to take suspected cases to treatment centres, quarantining their families, tracing their contacts, and conducting house-to-house searches for hidden cases. All this hard work paid off and by mid-April the outbreak was over. However, one Aberdeen fisherman who had been quarantined when the first cases of Ebola appeared in the township decided to head home to his village when he became unwell. He escaped quarantine by hiding in the back of a truck and managed to pass at least a dozen check points before arriving in Rosanda, a village some 200km from Aberdeen. Here he was cared for by his family for several days before dying of Ebola.

Large numbers gathered for his funeral, many of whom participated in the ritual washing of his body. According to some, the villagers then drank the washings; be that as it may, they reportedly washed in the contaminated water and poured it over themselves, leaving the village children to play in the Ebola-infested puddles. Twenty-four people, both children and adults, contracted Ebola at this funeral. Nevertheless, having witnessed what Ebola could do, thereafter villagers cooperated willingly with health care workers and the chains of infection set in motion at the funeral were soon terminated.

The second incident was in Moa Wharf;[11] another of Freetown's seaside slums where Ebola raged first in March 2014 and then again in April 2015. This second wave of Ebola was unusual in targeting mainly young men. The death rate was particularly high because sufferers hid in the community. The index case turned out to be a member of a secret club called the Black Star Liner Three Poli Boys, named after a fishing boat wrecked in coastal waters nearby. The boys in the secret club ate, slept, smoked, and drank together, but tracing club members proved impossible. Because of their anti-social behaviour the boys were outcasts in the township; no one wanted to talk about them and so the Ebola response team was met by a wall of silence. Knowing that they were in danger of developing Ebola, the boys simply melted away, believing that 'once they take you away, you never come back'. But one by one they became too sick to hide and were taken into isolation. Yet, at some point there was a transformation; MSF workers managed to enlist the help of the remaining boys in contact tracing and case finding. Once it became clear that the boys were helping with the fight against Ebola, the community forgave their past misdemeanours. Eventually, wearing 'Kick Ebola Out' T-shirts, the boys became leaders in the 'We Will Beat It' campaign in Moa Wharf.

6

~~

Ebola Epidemic

The Endgame

The fight against Ebola had lasted well over a year by the time it reached its endgame in summer 2015. As the number of cases fell, the epidemic dropped out of the headlines and most people either lost interest or assumed that it was already over. In West Africa, several NGOs packed up and left, while the staff of those remaining were simply exhausted. Tired, grieving communities in the three worst affected countries just wanted life to return to normal, and a kind of communal lethargy set in. Concerned, Joanna Liu, MSF International President, said: 'On Ebola, we went from global indifference, to global fear, to global response and now global fatigue. We must finish the job.'[1]

Liu's fear was exemplified by figures from MSF workers in Guinea showing that even after all the effort expended on community engagement, 25% of Ebola cases were still being concealed in the community and only discovered by the authorities after death. With hindsight, and viewed from the perspective of the afflicted population, these figures were understandable. 'In the Ebola epidemic, strangers showed up in villages in what looked like space suits and took away loved ones, with only around half being seen again. At the peak of the epidemic, people were often not told when their relatives had died or were not given the chance to bury their dead according to custom,' says Liu.[2] The epidemic would not end until *all* cases were declared and isolated. It was imperative to retain the capacity built up in phases 1 and 2 of the response while doubling efforts in phase 3 until the job was done.[3]

Phase 3 had two main objectives—*achieving and sustaining a resilient zero.* The first objective meant defining and rapidly interrupting all remaining chains of Ebola transmission. While this sounds like more of the same, it had some important, new, scaled-up and improved activities over the phase 2 response. WHO had learned lessons from the many challenging situations their teams faced during phase 2, the implications of which formed the basis of the phase 3 plans. The following descriptions of two Ebola outbreaks in Liberia illustrate the difficulties encountered in remote areas—poor transport and communications infrastructure as well as community resistance to essential intervention measures.[4]

In late 2014, Ebola was introduced to several remote villages in Liberia by travellers from Ebola-affected areas, usually Monrovia, returning to their homes. One such outbreak occurred in Geleyansiesu, a village in Gbarpolu County with around 800 inhabitants and only accessible by canoe along the Saint Paul River followed by several hours' walk. The index case was a 10-year-old girl who returned from school in Kakata, Margibi County, on September 16. She became ill on September 18 and died at home on September 27. This set an Ebola transmission trail in motion that included first her stepmother and then her father. The Bong County Health Team was only alerted to the situation in late October when the father was admitted to a treatment centre. The team visited Geleyansiesu along with experts from CDC and other international partners, but found no Ebola cases. However, villagers *did* report the recent deaths of two farmers, one apparently from accidental injuries. Neither farmer had links with the index case so it seemed possible that the virus transmission trail had run its course. Nevertheless, the team educated villagers about Ebola symptoms and treatment, case investigation, contact tracing and monitoring, and provided training in safe burials. They also taught villagers how to isolate and give limited, no-touch treatment to Ebola sufferers who were unable to reach a treatment centre.

Because of the village's complete lack of telecommunications, the team posted a Bong County Health Official at the Saint Paul River crossing—the closest vehicle access point to the village. This team member could then provide regular updates back to base via mobile phone and also arrange transport to the nearest Ebola treatment centre for any sick villagers able to walk to the river crossing. In fact, seven sick villagers, all family members of the dead farmers, reached the access point on November 3. They were admitted to Bong treatment centre where they all tested positive for Ebola and five died. These were followed by another six Ebola cases, also contacts of the farmers either before or after death, five of whom died.

The investigating team returned to Geleyansiesu on November 9 and uncovered six more probable Ebola cases. They set up an isolation tent in the village for two cases unable to walk to the access point but both refused to move and died in their own homes. Ten days later the team again visited the village to assess the situation but were forced to leave after encountering hostility from a group of villagers. They then contacted the district's paramount chief (the traditional leader) who facilitated a peaceful visit. No new

Ebola cases were found during this visit and the outbreak was declared over on December 20, 2014. There had been a total of twenty-two Ebola cases and sixteen deaths.

Another Ebola outbreak in the similar-sized village of Mawah, Bong County, was again sparked by a student returning to his home village. He was already sick when he arrived in Mawah on August 31 and he died on September 4 and was buried by family members. A second villager, a contact of the index case, fell ill on September 9 and died of Ebola. The County Health Team quarantined six families that had had contact with him and/or the index case, and between September 17 and 20 six more villagers died of Ebola. At this stage the team proposed a community quarantine period of twenty-one days. In practical terms this meant establishing check points on access roads to prevent anyone entering or leaving the village, closing local markets, and regulating the Saint Paul River crossing near the village. Discussions with local leaders identified two concerns about this plan. First, it would leave villagers without a supply of food and unable to earn an income since their livelihood depended on fishing in the river and growing rice in paddies on the opposite river bank. Second, as the Mawah health clinic had closed down during the Ebola epidemic, the nearest health services were in a neighbouring village that would be inaccessible during the proposed quarantine period. Nevertheless, community quarantine *was* imposed on October 1, with assurances that the village clinic would reopen for two days a week and food aid would be provided. But although the World Food Programme agreed to deliver food rations for forty-five days, and a nurse equipped with a contactless thermometer was promised for the clinic, neither the food nor the nurse arrived in the village for a week after instigation of quarantine.

Unsurprisingly, these delays caused resentment among villagers, as did the plan to regulate the river crossing. It was finally agreed that farmers could cross the river to their paddies each morning and return in the evening. Two canoe pilots were nominated to ferry them across while all other canoes were chained to trees. Hand washing at the crossing was obligatory and pilots were instructed not to transport non-residents or sick villagers. Fortunately, after the County Health Team accompanied by CDC officials inspected the village on October 1 and arranged for transportation of twenty-four suspected Ebola cases to a treatment centre in Monrovia, no further cases occurred. When quarantine was lifted on October 31 there had been twenty-two cases and nineteen deaths among Mawah residents.

With these difficult management issues in mind, the emphasis in phase 3 was on coordinating multidisciplinary, quick-response teams including epidemiologists, anthropologists, contact tracers, social mobilization, and other experts, all under national leadership. Teams would assess, implement, manage, and monitor the response to each 'event'—meaning each new transmission trail. Gaining the trust of community leaders was paramount to the success of this plan and so sufficient personnel had to be assigned to each event investigation to allow for these, sometimes lengthy, interactions. Time had to be spent educating communities about Ebola transmission, symptoms, patient isolation, and the benefits of early diagnosis and treatment. Only then could community leaders take responsibility for identifying and monitoring case contacts, tracing missing contacts (even continuing the search after twenty-one days to determine the contacts' state of health), managing quarantined households, and performing safe, dignified burials. Listening to and addressing the concerns of communities and their leaders was essential for gaining full cooperation, something that had often not been a priority in the past, particularly in difficult-to-reach communities like Geleyansiesu and Mawah, where circumstances beyond the control of visiting health teams allowed Ebola to gain the upper hand.

To pre-empt village leaders' concerns regarding quarantine orders, as experienced in Mawah, a 'package' of aid would be offered up front to each community. This had to be individualized to the villagers' specific needs, and would include incentives to encourage case contacts to come forward and for the community as a whole to cooperate. Any of the following might be included: food, clean water, sanitation and hygiene, protection of livelihoods, and psycho-social support for recovered cases and bereaved families. Reactivation of primary health services that had been closed at the height of the Ebola epidemic was clearly important so that antenatal care, routine vaccinations, and treatment of common diseases other than Ebola could resume.

Immediate genetic sequencing of viruses isolated from all Ebola cases was part of the phase 3 plan, in order to accurately identify the source of the virus in each case. This would rapidly unravel complex transmission chains and avoid delays in estimating individual risks for family members and contacts of Ebola cases. As described earlier, when the team of investigators arrived in Geleyansiesu village, they thought that the risk of onward transmission was low because the trail set in motion by the index case seemed to have run its course. However, a cluster of new cases arose among villagers who had no links with the index case but *were* contacts of the two dead farmers. Later genetic analysis made sense of this puzzle by revealing that there had been two separate introductions of Ebola into the village virtually simultaneously;

one by the schoolgirl and the other by one of the farmers. If this information had been available at the time then tracing and isolation of the farmers' contacts could have cut this transmission chain short.

Vaccination against, and drug treatment for, Ebola was a completely new aspect of the phase 3 plan, made possible at this late stage in the epidemic because candidate vaccines and drugs that were in development when the epidemic began were now ready for testing in the field. Details of these products, their development, and clinical trials, are covered in Chapter 8, but a stated priority in the phase 3 plan was implementing vaccination for contacts and contacts-of-contacts.[5] The possibility of preventing the awful suffering caused by Ebola, and the high likelihood of death, by a simple course of injections must surely have been a strong incentive for family members and contacts of Ebola cases to come forward for vaccination.

*   *   *

Implementation of the first objective of the phase 3 plan—*to define and rapidly interrupt all remaining chains of Ebola transmission*—led to the WHO Ebola-free declaration and accompanying celebrations in Liberia on May 9, 2015, after having had no new Ebola cases for forty-two days (twice the incubation period). The country then entered a three-month period of heightened surveillance during which around thirty samples daily—blood and mouth swabs from potential cases—were tested for Ebola. Just seven weeks later, one of these samples—from a 17-year-old youth from Nedowein village, near Monrovia—tested positive. He had died on June 28 and his post mortem blood tested Ebola positive on June 29—the first confirmed case of Ebola in Liberia since March 20. This spawned a cluster of five cases from the same village, with two deaths. Genetic analysis of viruses recovered from the victims showed that the infections constituted a single transmission chain, and suggested that the index case's infection arose by re-emergence of the virus contracted from a survivor rather than the introduction of a new strain.[6]

On September 3, 2015, Liberia again celebrated the end of its fifteen-month long Ebola epidemic after having no new Ebola cases for another forty-two days. However, on November 22, a 15-year-old boy with Ebola was admitted to a treatment centre in Monrovia where he died. This case was again caused by re-emergence of the virus from a survivor and spawned a cluster of three cases including the boy's father and brother.

Sierra Leone was confirmed Ebola free on November 7, Guinea on December 29, 2015, and finally Liberia for the third time on January 14, 2016. At this point WHO declared the epidemic over and reported the final figures as 28,637 cases and 11,315 deaths, with 3,804 cases and 2,536 deaths in Guinea, 14,122 cases and 3,955 deaths in Sierra Leone, and 10,672 cases and 4,808 deaths in Liberia (Figure 11). Overall the death rate for the epidemic was 40% but locally this figure varied considerably depending on the availability of supportive treatment.

Fantastic as these Ebola-free declarations were they did not mean that all international support teams could pack up and go home. Both national and international teams still had plenty of work to do in identifying, and responding to the consequences of, residual Ebola risks—the second objective of the phase 3 plan. In reality this meant maintaining the infrastructure to rapidly identify new Ebola cases. Swift notification and testing of all possible cases and suspicious deaths was essential, with immediate follow-up of positive results by multi-disciplinary Rapid Response Teams.

Weekly reported Ebola cases

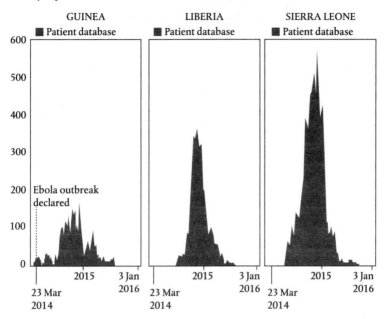

Figure 11 Graphs Showing Ebola cases in Guinea, Liberia, and Sierra Leone, 2014–16.

Indeed since January 2016 Ebola cases have been identified in all three countries but these have been quickly dealt with and the virus contained.

* * *

Little was known about the status of the virus in Ebola survivors at the start of the epidemic in West Africa, although the fact that male survivors could continue to produce infectious virus in semen for up to seven weeks after recovery was first established by a single case following the Yambuku outbreak in 1976. Studies from Kikwit, DRC, in 1995 and from Gulu District, Uganda, in 2000, identified infectious virus in blood and all bodily fluids during the acute

121

disease, but while most fluids became virus negative along with blood as soon as the acute stage of the disease was over, PCR detection of virus genome sequences remained positive for 101 days in semen.[7] However, virus amplification by PCR does not necessarily equate with *infectious* virus because a positive test can result from detection of non-infectious fragments of the virus genome. Nevertheless, in one study isolation of infectious virus from semen was possible for up to 82 days after onset of symptoms, raising the question of sexual transmission of Ebola virus disease.[8]

With these results in mind, CDC and WHO at first recommended that recovered Ebola sufferers always use a condom, which must be disposed of safely, or to abstain from sexual intercourse for at least three months. In addition, the phase 3 plan proposed screening and counselling all male survivors for at least three months after recovery, and, if necessary, monthly thereafter until semen samples had twice tested Ebola negative. Then, a study undertaken during the 2014–16 Ebola epidemic, detected virus genome in semen from male survivors for up to nine months after disease onset,[9] and at the same time convincing evidence of sexual transmission of Ebola virus came to light.[10]

On March 20, 2015, thirty days after the previous Ebola case in Liberia had been diagnosed, a 44-year-old woman from Monrovia developed the disease. She died on March 27. When questioned she denied any contact with suspected or confirmed Ebola cases, had not recently attended a funeral, and gave no history of travelling to, or meeting with visitors from, Sierra Leone or Guinea. However, she *did* report having unprotected sexual intercourse with an Ebola survivor seven days before the onset of her symptoms. This male survivor, also from Monrovia, had developed Ebola on September 9, 2014, and was admitted to a treatment centre.

He was discharged on October 7, after which he was symptom free. Since his recovery he had had unprotected sexual intercourse with another woman on several occasions, but she remained well and tested Ebola negative. A semen sample collected from the survivor on March 27, 2015, tested PCR positive for Ebola, but two samples obtained at later dates were negative, as were all blood samples taken on the same dates. Thus his semen was Ebola virus positive 199 days after he developed symptoms of the disease.

Determining whether the female patient acquired Ebola by sexual transmission from the male survivor required comparison of RNA genome sequences of Ebola virus isolates from each individual. However, although routine PCR amplification procedures provided a complete genome sequence from the blood of the patient, it proved extremely difficult to extract Ebola virus RNA from the survivor's one Ebola positive semen sample. Eventually, scientists managed to sequence 85% of his virus genome to compare with the patient's virus RNA sequence. The results were conclusive. RNA sequences from the two Ebola viruses were virtually identical, only differing by one nucleotide in 85% of the 15,808 nucleotide-long Ebola genome available for comparison. In contrast, these virus genomes differed markedly from those obtained from the most recent Ebola cases in Liberia, which, since January 2015, had all been linked in a single transmission chain.[11]

As noted earlier, PCR detection of Ebola virus sequences does not prove that the virus is infectious, but in this case the additional molecular evidence of sexual transmission from survivor to patient was compelling and the implications were immense. It was now clear that reactivation of Ebola transmission could occur in the community well after the forty-two-day period that WHO allowed before declaring the danger of infection over.

This revelation, and the fact that the duration of viral persistence in semen was still unknown, led WHO to update the advice given to Ebola survivors,[12] now additionally recommending:

- counselling for all Ebola survivors and their sexual partners;
- regular Ebola testing of semen from Ebola survivors until two negative results are obtained;
- provision of condoms to survivors with advice to use them or abstain from sex completely until semen tests negative on two consecutive occasions. If a survivor's semen is not tested for Ebola then they should use condoms or abstain from sex for six months;
- observing good hand and personal hygiene by immediately and thoroughly washing with soap and water after physical contact with semen. Used condoms should be handled and disposed of safely, so as to prevent contact with seminal fluids.

* * *

The Ebola epidemic in West Africa produced over 17,000 Ebola survivors who face many challenges. The physical health of survivors was rarely studied in earlier outbreaks, although the few existing follow-up studies uncovered a multitude of problems. One report comparing Ebola survivors with case contacts who did not develop Ebola during the Bundibugyo outbreak in Uganda in 2007, found significantly more eye problems (pain and blurring of vision), hearing loss, joint pains, and difficulties in swallowing and in sleeping in the Ebola survivor group.[13] Similarly, eye and musculo-skeletal problems were identified among survivors of the Kikwit Ebola outbreak in 1995 and this constellation of symptoms has become known as the 'post-Ebola syndrome'. Like many post-viral symptoms, which may, for example, follow a bout of 'flu, and commonly include muscle and joint pains, headache, and lethargy, post-Ebola syndrome was thought to be immuno-pathological in nature. This means that the symptoms are caused by the body's own immune response to the virus rather than being due to damage caused by the virus persisting in the tissues. Following 'flu these symptoms fade in weeks, but at present we simply do not know the long-term outcome for sufferers of post-Ebola syndrome.

Because medical facilities and personnel were so overstretched at the height of the Ebola epidemic, no investigations into post-Ebola problems could be undertaken in West Africa until case numbers began to wane. But the few foreign health care workers who were repatriated after developing Ebola were fully investigated and on occasions these cases uncovered new and surprising results. Two such cases of severe post-Ebola complications were exhaustively studied and revealed new insights into the pathological mechanisms underlying Ebola virus disease and the post-Ebola syndrome.

Forty-three-year-old American physician Ian Crozier caught Ebola while working in the treatment centre at Kenema, Sierra Leone, in September 2014. Dubbed 'the sickest Ebola victim to survive',[14] he was repatriated to the US and admitted to Emory University Hospital in Atlanta, after which his life hung in the balance for several weeks. 'I don't remember anything after I walked in the hospital doors [on September 8, 2014] until I woke up in late September...I would have been dead in a week had I stayed in Kenema', he says.[15] He was treated with an experimental drug called TKM-Ebola (see Chapter 8) and Ebola convalescent plasma to combat the virus as well as 'aggressive supportive care' for multi-organ system failure.[16] When his lungs failed they were mechanically ventilated for twelve days and when his kidneys shut down he required dialysis for twenty-four days. Encephalitis rendered him unconscious, and when he woke up he suffered loss of short-term memory, word-finding difficulties, and deafness. He lost thirty pounds in weight, he had to learn to walk again and he had joint and muscle pains, but, after a ten-week stay, he finally left hospital well on the road to recovery.

Unfortunately, just a few weeks later Crozier experienced pain and blurred vision in his left eye and noticed that the colour of the iris had changed from blue to green. He was diagnosed with acute pan-uveitis—inflammation in the anterior and posterior chambers of the eye—an extremely painful condition that is sight-threatening if left untreated. The exact cause of this condition was unclear and so Crozier received anti-viral agents to kill the virus along with steroids to suppress inflammation, a drug combination that, thankfully, worked, and his sight was saved. But he was still left with many problems. 'I'm frustrated by the way my life has changed,' he says, 'I have an MRI [magnetic resonance imaging] full of holes, reflecting areas of my brain that have clearly been damaged. I can't run anymore and I get tired very easily.'[17]

While his eye problems were ongoing, samples of Crozier's blood and tears tested Ebola negative, indicating that there was no risk of virus spread to others. But fluid extracted from the anterior chamber of his left eye tested strongly positive for Ebola virus. Furthermore, successful culture of the virus from this fluid proved that it was infectious.

The second unique, repatriated, Ebola case was a 39-year-old Scottish nurse who caught the virus while working as a volunteer in Kerry Town treatment centre, Sierra Leone, in December 2014. She suffered severe Ebola virus disease and was admitted to the high-level isolation facility at the Royal Free Hospital, London, where she received experimental anti-viral drugs, convalescent plasma, and intensive supportive treatment. When she left the hospital twenty-eight days later no Ebola virus RNA was detectable in her blood and she was apparently cured of the disease. Even so, over the next few months she suffered joint pains and hair loss, and then, nine months after she left hospital, she fell gravely ill. She was admitted to hospital in Scotland complaining of headache, stiff neck, and photophobia and then swiftly transferred to the high-level isolation unit at the Royal Free Hospital where she was diagnosed with Ebola meningoencephalitis and said to be 'fighting for her life'.[18] This is the first case of Ebola meningoencephalitis ever recorded after recovery from the acute disease. The nurse was given supportive care and again treated with experimental drugs. She was eventually discharged from hospital some fifty-two days later having made a clinical recovery but still with some residual problems.[19] Dr Michael Jacobs, Infectious Diseases Consultant at the Royal Free Hospital said 'This is the original Ebola virus she had many months ago which has been inside her brain, replicating at a very low level, and has now re-emerged to cause this clinical illness of meningitis. This is an unprecedented situation.'[20] Because the nurse had infectious virus in her blood and cerebro-spinal fluid, fifty-eight of her contacts, including members of the Scottish medical team that first examined her, were offered Ebola vaccination and placed under surveillance. Fortunately, none developed Ebola.

Finding Ebola virus replicating in the testes, eyes, and central nervous system for long periods after recovery from the acute disease completely changes our understanding of the pathology of Ebola virus disease and post-Ebola syndrome. Right now these revelations raise more questions than they answer, but one thing is obvious—Ebola virus disease can no longer be regarded as a

typical acute infection after which the virus is completely eliminated from the body. Clearly some humans act as reservoirs of
Ebola virus, and although there may only be a few of these virus
carriers, and the risk of them transmitting the virus might be low,
nevertheless, such an event could kick start a new Ebola outbreak.
Large studies on Ebola survivors are now ongoing in West Africa
to detect all possible sites of virus sequestration in the body, to
define the duration of virus persistence, and to understand the
mechanisms used by the virus to avoid being wiped out by the
immune system. Only with this information to hand can we estimate the risk of, and devise measures to prevent, chronic virus
carriage and the consequent sparking of an Ebola outbreak.

The gonads, eyes, and central nervous system are all sites
known to harbour persistent viruses. Indeed, Ebola's close relative,
Marburg virus, can persist in the eye and has also been reported in
semen from some survivors, while certain herpes viruses commonly persist for life in the central nervous system and even the
measles virus can occasionally do so. These organs are called
sanctuary sites, or immune-privileged sites, because immune cells
cannot penetrate their tissues efficiently and so certain viruses
may survive there unharmed. This is also the case with the placenta and developing foetus in which replicating viruses such as
the rubella virus may cause tissue damage leading to congenital
abnormalities.

The physiological mechanisms underlying the exclusion of
immune cells from certain body sites are not fully understood and
may indeed vary between different organs. Virus persistence in
these sites is particularly likely if a patient's immune system is
weakened by a concurrent chronic infection such as HIV, ongoing
cancer chemotherapy, or a genetic immune defect that affects the

ability to clear viruses. Right now the state of Ebola virus in these sanctuary sites is unknown. It may be that the virus, like HIV and measles, is continuously replicating at a low level in the tissues, in which case it could continue to cause tissue damage. On the other hand, Ebola virus could enter a dormant state like that of herpes viruses, in which it is invisible to the immune system but can be reactivated by certain triggers that induce immune suppression to cause resurgent disease.

In the light of these new findings, the pathology underlying the headaches, fatigue, muscle and joint pains, and eye problems of post-Ebola syndrome, previously assumed to be an immune-pathological condition, must be reassessed. Since live virus was recovered from cases of uveitis and meningitis, it is also possible that virus replication is responsible for post-Ebola symptoms reported in around 40% of survivors of the 2014–16 Ebola epidemic. These survivors are still suffering and face an uncertain future. They are not as fortunate as Crozier and the Scottish nurse; without support some may die of meningitis and others lose their sight. It is imperative that they get the help and support they need to ensure their future good health and that research into the cause of the syndrome continues with a view to preventing survivors becoming a source of infection.

* * *

The Ebola epidemic in West Africa caused immense psychological trauma,[21] and this was not restricted to just survivors of the disease. Thousands of people in the three worst affected countries were left grieving for lost relatives and friends while close to 10,000 children lost one parent and around 600 lost both their parents.[22] Many of the bereaved believed that because they had not given their dead relatives traditional burial rites the whole community was sick and consequently they have found it impossible to move on. Ebola survivors had additional problems with haunting memories, guilt for having caught the disease and, on occasion, stigmatization by their family, community, and/or work colleagues. Some were ostracized from their homes while others lost their livelihood. Fifty-eight-year-old English teacher Beatrice Yardolo, the last Ebola sufferer to recover in Liberia, lost two sons and a niece to Ebola. She vowed not to return to her teaching job because she said 'I am afraid that parents will complain about me teaching their children…I have decided to avoid this embarrassment.' Comparing the Ebola epidemic to the civil wars she witnessed in Liberia, Yardolo adds: 'It is easier to run away from guns in a war than from such an unseen enemy.'[23]

Prior to the Ebola epidemic in West Africa, mental health services in the region were at best rudimentary and often non-existent. Liberia was the only one of the three severely affected countries with a hospital dedicated to mental health (the E.S. Grant Mental Health Hospital in Monrovia), but even this hospital closed during the epidemic for fear of Ebola spreading from patients to health care workers. Most of the patients were discharged, compounding the mental health problem by forcing homeless, sick, and psychotic patients to wander the streets.

In the past, most psychological problems were treated by traditional healers, who likely succeeded in calming fears with their traditional herbal remedies. But the overwhelming post-Ebola problem required immediate support for sufferers as well as a long-term, sustainable solution to their plight. NGOs did what they could to relieve the situation with simple approaches such as portraying survivors as heroes to overcome the stigma of Ebola, offering bereaved families counselling and, where possible, providing photos of their deceased loved ones' bodies. Meanwhile, the World Bank, national and foreign governments, and NGOs have donated funds to build a mental health infrastructure in the three countries by training psychiatric nurses and counsellors to provide psychological support to the victims. But with the present level of suspicion regarding Western medicine, doctors, and nurses, compounded by fear and distrust of authorities, it is essential to work with traditional healers and incorporate their methods if any plan for mental health services is to gain acceptance by the wider community.

* * *

Pregnant women suffered particularly cruelly during the epidemic.[24] As a group they are uniquely susceptible to Ebola, perhaps because of the natural immune suppression that occurs during pregnancy. Also, Ebola increases the likelihood of haemorrhage during childbirth which adds to the risk for both mother and child. Virtually no babies born to Ebola-infected mothers survive, and recent studies have uncovered the reason—Ebola virus in the mother's blood crosses the placenta to infect foetal tissues.[25]

Pregnant women with Ebola pose a serious threat to health care workers because of the infected blood and body fluids released during labour, and it is estimated that around a third of care workers who died of Ebola in the first six months of the epidemic worked in maternity wards. Seeing the risk, many others deserted their posts and those remaining were understandably terrified of caring for pregnant women. The dilemma was that the abdominal pain experienced in early stages of labour could be caused by Ebola and so Ebola testing was essential to distinguish between the two. But while Ebola testing took at least twenty-four hours, women in labour needed help immediately. So the only *safe* way to care for mothers in labour during the Ebola epidemic was to don full protective gear, although this restrictive clothing made it almost impossible to provide the care needed. As a result, pregnant women were often refused entry to Ebola clinics and treatment centres, some giving birth and dying with their babies alone on the floor of waiting rooms or in the back of ambulances. Hearing these horror stories, others opted to give birth at home, putting their family at high risk of catching the virus.

Either directly or indirectly, Ebola claimed several thousands of maternal deaths in Guinea, Sierra Leone, and Liberia. But its legacy is far greater—with the resulting lack of trained staff combined with mothers' loss of trust, the maternal death rate in the region, already unacceptably high, is projected to double to 1,000–2,000 per 100,000 in the coming years.

*   *   *

During 2014, the peak of the Ebola epidemic coincided with the height of the malaria season in Guinea and Sierra Leone. Many primary health care facilities had closed during the Ebola epidemic because, with close to 500 health care workers dead from Ebola, and those able to work redirected to the fight against the virus, there was no one to replace them. Even in the facilities that remained open during the crisis, patient attendance was low; in some cases just 10% of the expected level for the time of year.[26] Non-attendance was particularly common among patients with fever, who were afraid of either being diagnosed with Ebola and transferred to an isolation unit or of catching Ebola at the clinic.

Malaria is hyper-endemic in Guinea, Sierra Leone, and Liberia, meaning that it is transmitted (via mosquitoes) all year round. The disease particularly targets young children, and in this region of West Africa blood parasites are present in the blood of up to 44% of children under five years of age. In Liberia malaria transmission remains at a constant level throughout the year, while in Guinea and Sierra Leone the levels rise sharply each year during the rainy season between May and July.

In the past decade there has been a major push to tackle the problem of malaria in Sub Saharan Africa where approximately 90% of the annual global 500,000 deaths occur. A scaled-up intervention programme across the region has succeeded in reducing childhood mortality from malaria by around 50%. The mainstay of this intervention is insecticide-treated bed nets combined with indoor insecticide spraying to prevent bites from night-flying mosquitoes, as well as rapid malaria diagnosis and treatment for those presenting themselves at health care facilities with fever. In 2013, WHO reported 3.5 million malaria cases and 16,000 deaths in Guinea, 1.5 million cases with 7,800 deaths in Sierra Leone, and 371,500 cases with 2,419 deaths in Liberia.

We will probably never know exactly how many people lost their lives to malaria in Guinea, Sierra Leone, and Liberia during the Ebola epidemic in 2014–16. Certainly bednets, which deteriorate over time, were not widely distributed and many malaria cases went untreated. A small survey was undertaken in sixty health care facilities in four Ebola-affected and four Ebola-free prefectures in Guinea in December 2014. The results showed no difference between affected and unaffected prefectures but indicated that in 2014 the Ebola epidemic resulted in around 74,000 suspected malaria cases being left untreated countrywide.[27] In another study scientists used mathematical modelling to predict numbers for malaria cases and deaths in 2014 in the whole Ebola-affected area.[28] Several potential scenarios were modelled, but in the nightmare situation of malaria care ceasing completely, the model predicted 3.5 million additional malaria cases with 10,900 deaths.

These devastating predictions hint at the full extent of the humanitarian crisis caused by Ebola in West Africa. Clearly the epidemic had a far greater effect than the appalling morbidity and mortality caused by the disease itself. By suggesting that during 2014 numbers dying of malaria and of Ebola were comparable, the study highlights the plight of the non-Ebola-infected population in the epidemic area. What's more, considering that malaria is just one of a multitude of preventable and treatable infectious diseases rife in West Africa, we can expect to see a resurgence of TB, HIV, measles, polio, and many others before health services are reconstituted in the region.

On a more positive note, during the 2015 rainy season, and as the Ebola epidemic was diminishing, WHO recommended a mass drug administration programme. In practice this meant administering anti-malarial drugs to everyone, regardless of symptoms, in areas badly affected by Ebola and with high malaria transmission. The aim was to rapidly reduce deaths from malaria, to decrease the numbers reporting to community care and treatment centres with fever not caused by Ebola, thereby reducing the risk of Ebola transmission, and to improve the credibility of health care services in the affected countries.[29] The malaria modelling study looked forward to 2015 and predicted that if this mass drug administration and distribution of insecticide-impregnated bednets coincided with the peak malaria transmission between May and July 2015 this 'could substantially reduce additional malaria burden'.[30] This prediction was based on monthly drug administration and mass bednet distribution with 70% coverage. MSF implemented the plan in Freetown and Monrovia using an artesunate-amodiaquine drug combination that both treats and prevents malaria.[31] In the face of an ongoing Ebola epidemic this was a challenging undertaking, but although uptake of the drugs by families in both capital cities was very encouraging, contributing a welcome reduction in parasite transmission during the 2015 rainy season, many unnecessary malaria deaths still occurred in rural areas.

So once again, these collateral effects of the Ebola epidemic will continue well after the containment of the epidemic itself, their recovery depending critically on the rebuilding of both health services and community trust in them.

7

2014 Ebola Epidemic

Where, When, and How?

In trying to uncover where and when the Ebola epidemic began, medical detectives set about tracing contacts of the earliest reported cases in Guékédou and Macenta prefectures in southeastern Guinea. By following chains of infection back through suspected cases and their contacts, affected families, and villages, the team quickly revealed evidence that the virus had been in the area for quite some time before the Ebola cases came to light.[1] So although the *apparent* beginning of the outbreak was in March 2014, the timeline of events constructed by the team pinpointed December 2013 as the beginning of the outbreak and Meliandou, a small village of just thirty-one houses surrounded by farm land in the prefecture of Guékédou, as ground zero. The virus spread from here to the prefectures of Macenta and Kissidougou, all within the three months prior to the alert being sent to the Guinean Ministry of Health on March 10, 2014 (Figure 12).

In December 2013 a 2-year-old boy in Meliandou called Emile Ouamouno became ill with fever, vomiting, and bloody diar-

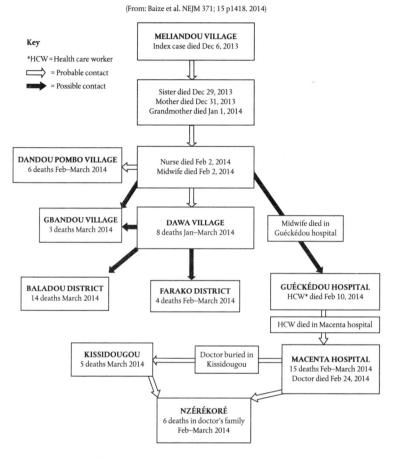

EARLY TRANSMISSION CHAINS IN THE OUTBREAK OF EBOLA VIRUS DISEASE IN GUINEA 2013-2014

(From: Baize et al. NEJM 371; 15 p1418. 2014)

Figure 12   Flowchart of first Ebola cases in Guinea, 2013–14.

rhoea. He died on December 6. His pregnant mother then became unwell. She suffered a miscarriage with excessive bleeding and died on December 13. Emile's 3-year-old sister Philomène then came down with diarrhoea and vomiting and died on December 29, followed by their grandmother on January 1, 2014. During their illnesses the Ouamouno family had been tended by the village nurse and the midwife, both of whom developed the same disease. While the nurse died at home on February 2 without infecting anyone else, the Meliandou village midwife became an Ebola super-spreader. First she carried the virus to Gbandou village, where at least three people died of the disease in early March. When she became ill she was cared for by her family in her home village of Dandou Pombo where, during February and March 2014 six deaths occurred. The sick midwife was eventually admitted to hospital in Guéckédou on January 25 and died eight days later. A health care worker in the hospital who probably caught the virus from her, started a chain of infection that carried the virus to the prefectures of Nzerekore, Kissidougou, and also Macenta where she was admitted to hospital and died on February 10.

Meanwhile, in Meliandou, a crowd gathered for Emile's grandmother's funeral that included her sister and a friend, both from Dawa village. They assisted in the traditional burial rituals and both developed Ebola after returning home to Dawa. The women died in late January 2014. The virus spread from them to Gbandou village (for a second time) and had also reached Guéckédou Baladou District and Guéckédou Farako District by the end of February. From this focus the virus established chains of infection that travelled relentlessly onwards in an ever-growing wave.

The death rate for these very first, unrecognized cases was 86% but by the time the disease was finally diagnosed as Ebola on March 22, 2014, there had been 111 suspected cases and seventy-nine deaths—a fatality rate of 71%. Interestingly, at this stage almost all the Ebola cases were women and the haemorrhagic symptoms that generally characterize Ebola disease were relatively unusual. Instead patients more commonly suffered from fever, vomiting, and severe diarrhoea—non-specific symptoms that make Ebola so difficult to diagnose without laboratory backup.

* * *

Since no virus transmission chain leading to 2-year-old Emile Ouamouno could be uncovered, he was the presumed index case for the whole outbreak. So the question then became—how did Emile pick up the virus? This was addressed by a group of German scientists who undertook a four-week field study in Guéckédou in April 2014.[2] The group knew that several previous Ebola outbreaks, including the only human Ebola infection ever recorded in West Africa (in Côte d'Ivoire in 1994), resulted from virus transmission from chimpanzees and gorillas. So first they carried out a survey of non-human primates in the area. Although these species are rare in southeastern Guinea, the team found no evidence of a further decline in their numbers or of recently discovered carcasses in the forest. Furthermore, local villagers said that they rarely hunted large game; mostly they consumed imported, smoked primate meat from northeastern Guinea and Liberia. Also, if primate meat had been the source of the outbreak, then it seems likely that the index case would have been a hunter or member of a hunter's family, while Emile's father was a farmer. On this basis the team ruled out large game as the origin of the outbreak and concentrated their attention on the presumed animal reservoir of Ebola—bats. Men in Meliandou and surrounding villages admitted to catching and eating bats whenever they could. Local hunters described caves inhabited by colonies of fruit bats and also reported regular migrations of large numbers of these bats into the area. But more striking was the information that insect-eating bats, which commonly live under roofs or in hollow trees, were regularly hunted by village children, then grilled over small fires and eaten. With this news the team set about catching and testing these local bats, including species which had previously tested positive for Ebola, but none of more than 100 bats tested showed evidence of Ebola.

Finally, villagers pointed out a large, burnt tree stump on the edge of the village some 50m (55 yards) from Emile's home. This was the remains of a hollow tree that had been a favourite haunt of village children who often trapped and played with the bats that roosted in it. The tree had burnt down in March 2014 and as it burnt a 'rain of bats' began. The villagers caught these bats with the intention of eating them, but the very next day the Guinean Government banned consumption of bush meat and so they disposed of their catch. On hearing this story the team collected ash and soil samples from around the burnt tree stump to test for bat DNA. Five of eleven samples tested positive for DNA of the Angolan free-tailed bat (*Mops condylurus*), a common insect-eating bat in southeastern Guinea. Since this bat species had previously tested positive for Ebola antibodies,[3] the team thought this the most likely source of Emile's Ebola virus, however, this theory remains circumstantial.

* * *

With continued exponential rise of Ebola cases in West Africa for over eight months in 2014, experts worried that the virus responsible for this outbreak could be a mutated, more virulent form than the viruses that caused previous outbreaks. To address this concern a team from WHO collected detailed clinical information on the behaviour of the virus and the nature of the disease it caused during the first nine months of the epidemic to compare with data from previous outbreaks. This confirmed earlier reports suggesting that bleeding was an unusual symptom, only being reported in up to 6% of cases, while the more common symptoms of fever, fatigue, headache, loss of appetite, vomiting, abdominal pain, and diarrhoea remained the same as on previous occasions.[4] The overall death rate at this stage was around 70% in all three countries, but was consistently lower, at around 64%, for hospitalized patients. Risk factors for a fatal outcome included age over 45 years, difficulty in breathing or swallowing, diarrhoea, conjunctivitis, bleeding, and central nervous system symptoms such as disorientation and coma. The average incubation period was 11.4 days and average time between hospital admission and death was four days, or twelve days to discharge from hospital for those who recovered. Estimates of the basic reproductive number, R_0, at this early stage were 1.7 for Guinea, 2.02 for Sierra Leone, and 1.2 for Liberia, indicating that the epidemic was still growing in all three countries. All these statistics from the ongoing epidemic, including the all-important R_0 value, were similar to those of previous outbreaks in their early stages, prompting WHO to conclude: 'that the present epidemic is exceptionally large, not principally because of the biological characteristics of the virus, but rather because of the attributes of the affected populations and because control efforts have been insufficient to halt spread of infection.'

This conclusion was corroborated by other studies comparing RNA sequences of several hundred Ebola viruses isolated from early cases. These showed that the Ebola virus was changing at the expected, natural evolutionary rate. Furthermore, there was no change in mutation rate over the course of the epidemic and no mutations were identified that might increase transmissibility of the virus.[5] These combined clinical and molecular studies allayed fears that the unprecedented size of the ongoing epidemic was due to a mutated Ebola virus with increased virulence and/or rate of spread in humans.

It might have been expected that the offending virus in the 2014–16 epidemic was *Tai Forest ebolavirus*—a virus strain previously isolated in Côte d'Ivoire, a country that borders both Guinea and Liberia. But Ebola genome sequencing projects came up with some surprising news. The culprit was rapidly identified as *Zaire ebolavirus*, the virus first isolated during the Yambuku outbreak in 1976 and which thereafter had only caused outbreaks in DRC and Gabon.[6] The very close similarity between genome sequences of virus isolates from Ebola cases in early 2014 confirmed that the epidemic was sparked by a single introduction of *Zaire ebolavirus* into humans, but also showed that this virus was sufficiently different from all other known *Zaire ebolavirus* viruses to constitute a new virus strain. This is now called the *Makona virus strain* after the Makona River, which runs close to Meliandou village where the first Ebola cases occurred, and scientists have unravelled its fascinating history.

The genome of the Makona virus strain differs from that of *Zaire ebolavirus* strains from DRC and Gabon by 3%, enough to show that it did not evolve directly from these strains. At its natural evolution rate Ebola virus would take around ten years to accumulate a 3% change in genome sequence, so the only explanation was that the Makona virus strain had evolved in parallel with the DRC and Gabon viruses, diverging from common stock around 2004.[7] Thus, the Macona virus strain was not introduced directly into Guinea from either DRC or Gabon (and neither was it transported *to* DRC to cause the concurrent outbreak in Buende district, as some people had suggested). This rather surprising information implies that the Makona virus had been circulating undetected in West Africa for up to ten years before the 2014 outbreak began, most probably carried by bats or other animals that serve as an Ebola virus reservoir in the area.

Such findings were not arrived at without casualties. One of the publications reporting these genome studies ends with the following in memoriam: 'Tragically, five co-authors, who contributed greatly to public health and research efforts in Sierra Leone, contracted EVD [Ebola virus disease] and lost their battle with the disease before this manuscript could be published.'[8]

* * *

Several research groups used Ebola genome sequences to track the movements of the virus in the early stages of the outbreak in 2014. In general, virus genomes mutate around a million times faster than human DNA, and those with RNA genomes, like Ebola, evolve particularly rapidly. Mutations result from mistakes that occur when virus genomes are copied during the replication process. Offspring of a single virus will carry these sequence changes and so will have recognizably different genomes from the parent virus. Each time the offspring multiply they retain these original mutations while accumulating more. During epidemics viruses multiply quickly and so their genomes accumulate mutations rapidly. These form recognizable signatures that can be used to track their offspring along transmission chains. Using this so-called 'molecular epidemiology' alongside the more traditional epidemiological methods of case and case contact tracing, scientists uncovered the details of Ebola's uncharted spread from Guinea to Sierra Leone and Liberia (and back again) before effective case and contact finding was initiated.[9]

Key to Ebola's jump from Guinea to Sierra Leone and Liberia were the leaky borders between the three countries. Precisely at the epicentre of the outbreak in Guinea is an intersection where Guéckédou prefecture abuts Lofa County in Liberia and Kailahun district in Sierra Leone. In this remote forest region the local Kissi people refer to these international boundaries as 'open borders'. For them crossing the imaginary lines in the forest, on foot, by canoe, or motorcycle, to hunt, trade, or visit friends and family is an everyday occurrence. So by March 2014 Ebola was present in all three countries in this region and by early May it had reached Conakry, capital of Guinea. Interestingly, just one virus introduction from Guinea to Liberia and one from Guinea to Sierra Leone, took root and spread to cause outbreaks in those two countries. In contrast to these single introductions, the virus crossed back to Guinea from Liberia and Sierra Leone on several occasions so fuelling the epidemic in Guinea.

Ebola entered Liberia, in late March 2014, just as experts from CDC arrived in Guinea to assess the growing Ebola outbreak and assist in its management. But in May these experts returned home confident that everything was under control and the outbreak would soon be over. At this stage Ebola case numbers were dwindling in Conakry, and in Liberia cases dried up completely in April so that by the beginning of May twenty-one days had passed without a new case. Officials and experts assumed that this outbreak, like all past Ebola outbreaks, was responding to the classic control measures, and were optimistic that the end was in sight.

The first Ebola cases in Sierra Leone were confirmed in May 2014. But the virus had been spreading silently between villagers in Kailahun district, well before this date. As in villages across the border in Guinea, these early cases were cared for at home, often treated by traditional healers. Unsurprisingly then, several traditional healers became Ebola super-spreaders, inadvertently amplifying virus spread. One such was Finda Nyuma from Kpondu,

Kailahun district, who had treated several patients from nearby Guinea and Liberia with Ebola-like symptoms before dying of the same disease in early April. She was given a traditional funeral attended by hundreds of mourners, which generated several chains of infection. One of these led directly to Kenema Government Hospital where the first Ebola case in Sierra Leone was confirmed on May 24.[10] Molecular evidence shows that this was the only time the virus jumped from Guinea to Sierra Leone, with all subsequent cases in the country stemming from this single introduction.

In Liberia, the first wave of Ebola cases had completely died out in May, but just as treatment centres were being decontaminated and dismantled, a second wave hit the capital, Monrovia. This new outbreak was ignited by virus from cases on the Liberia–Sierra Leone border via the funeral of traditional healer Mendinor. She lived in Sierra Leone but regularly treated people on both sides of the border. She visited several presumed Ebola cases in the area before dying of the disease herself in May 2014. At her well-attended, traditional funeral at least thirteen women caught the virus and established transmission chains that not only fuelled the outbreak in Sierra Leone and Guinea but also initiated the second wave of infections in Monrovia, and this time the virus spread uncontrollably throughout the capital city and beyond.

With hindsight it is obvious that when CDC experts left Guinea in May satisfied that case numbers were dropping, and that the outbreak was largely confined to one country and was 'relatively small still'[11] they made a fatal error of judgement. Indeed, the outbreak in Liberia *had* died out, but only temporarily. Another took its place almost immediately, kindled from a quite different source. At this stage there had been just 383 cases and 211 deaths in the three countries. *If* the experts had stayed to oversee the effective implementation of the classic WHO guidelines for dealing with an Ebola outbreak then it would almost certainly have been contained. But the epidemic raged for another two months before WHO declared a Public Health Emergency of International Concern in August 2014, by which time case numbers were growing exponentially and the situation was completely out of control.

8

~~

Preventing Ebola

It is fair to speculate that if an effective vaccine against Ebola had been available prior to 2014, then once the initial outbreak in Guinea was recognized as such, virus spread could have been halted and many lives saved. Likewise, if there had been anti-Ebola drugs ready for use in the 2014–16 epidemic, this would have dramatically cut the death rate and curtailed the spread of the virus. Sadly, this was not the case. But there were high hopes that the epidemic would provide a unique opportunity to test anti-Ebola agents in those exposed to, or already infected with, the virus.

Broadly speaking there are two ways of combating infectious diseases; either preventing them with vaccines or using drugs to kill the offending microbes once they have taken hold. First pioneered by Edward Jenner at the end of the eighteenth century, smallpox vaccine was instrumental in ridding the world of the worst killer virus ever known. Now, in the twenty-first century, we have an arsenal of vaccines against disease-causing microbes that provides the mainstay of our global fight against infections. The general strategy is to induce 'herd immunity' by vaccinating at least 80% of a population.

This proportion is sufficient to prevent the microbes from circulating among members of the population, thereby protecting everyone from infection. Success of this approach means that many previously common, childhood infectious diseases, such as whooping cough, mumps, and rubella, are now rare in the West, while measles and polio viruses are well on the way to global extinction.

In a different vein, discovery of the first antibiotic, penicillin, by Alexander Fleming in the late 1920s, and its development by Howard Florey and colleagues in the 1940s, spawned a large family of drugs that kill or inactivate bacteria, such as those that cause pneumonia, meningitis, and typhoid fever. Unfortunately, antibiotics are ineffective against viruses because their mode of action involves attacking the bacterial cell wall, while viruses are inert particles that do not have cell walls. The development of anti-viral drugs only took off in the early 1980s in response to the global spread of HIV. Still not as numerous or as broadly effective as antibiotics for bacterial infections, anti-viral drugs tend to have restricted activity, targeting single or related virus families.

*   *   *

Development of a new drug or vaccine from its inception to its licensing for clinical use is a lengthy process that begins in the laboratory but also includes testing in a suitable animal model followed by clinical trials in humans. All this is extremely expensive and time-consuming, often taking ten or more years to complete. So, although the initial work may be conducted in a research institute or university department, collaboration with, and financial backing from, a commercial pharmaceutical company is generally needed to complete the job. Since commercial companies require a financial return from their investment, development and production of Ebola-specific drugs and vaccines has not been seen as a viable option. The reality is that prior to 2014, Ebola only caused small outbreaks that had always been fairly easily contained by following the classic WHO guidelines of case isolation, contact tracing, and safe burials. In fact, Ebola had killed a total of just 1,590 people since its discovery in 1976, so the likelihood of a large Ebola epidemic seemed very remote indeed.

At the end of the twentieth century, production of Ebola-specific agents was just a pipe dream, but one momentous event swung the odds in favour of Ebola vaccine and drug development. This was the memorable 9/11 terrorist attack in the US in 2001. As discussed in Chapter 2, the atrocity acted as a wake-up call for US and European governments to the threat of international bio-terrorism. Ebola disease virus is high on the list of candidate bio-weapons, and could possibly be manufactured and released by terrorist organizations. So, for the first time, Ebola prevention and treatment became a priority in the West. The aim was to produce drugs to treat any initial Ebola cases resulting from release of the virus, and to manufacture vaccines that would protect case contacts, health care workers, and those in the danger area, preferably after just a single shot. Ideally, a vaccine should also afford post-exposure protection, that is, prevent the disease even if administered after virus infection—a tall order, but nevertheless a feasible one.

When the epidemic began in 2014 several Ebola vaccines and drugs were in the pipeline although none was licensed for use in humans or ready for human trials. Even so, a number had been shown to be safe and effective in non-human primates and a few had already been manufactured to the standard required for human trials. Ideally, these potentially useful products should have passed all the time-consuming testing and legal processes required for clinical trials to proceed and been ready and waiting to test in the field as soon as the next Ebola outbreak occurred. In fact most had been shelved at an earlier stage of production due to lack of financial support for completing the job. So, frustratingly, although several potentially useful products existed, none was absolutely ready to go on day one of the epidemic.

Traditionally, once the efficacy of a new drug or vaccine has been demonstrated in an appropriate animal model, it has to go through a series of trials in humans (summarized in Table 2). First is a phase I trial that involves administering the product to around 20–100 volunteers to assess its safety, and determine the tolerated dose range. For a vaccine, a phase I trial also provides the opportunity to ascertain its ability to evoke an immune response in humans thereby providing protection against the microbe in question. Volunteers in a phase I trial are healthy adults, so for an Ebola-targeted agent this testing can be completed in the absence of an Ebola outbreak. If the results are favourable, then a phase II trial is conducted, generally recruiting several hundred participants to test efficacy and gather more information regarding the product's

Table 2 Summary of clinical trial phases

Phase	Design	Primary Goal	Dose	No. of Participants
Phase I	Open label, non-controlled	Safety	Ascending doses	20–100
Phase II	Randomized, controlled	Safety and efficacy	Therapeutic dose	100–300
Phase III	Double blind, randomized, controlled	Efficacy, effectiveness, and safety	Therapeutic dose	1,000–several thousand

safety. For the trial of a new *drug*, this requires volunteers who are suffering from the disease in question, but a phase II *vaccine* trial is conducted in volunteers at high risk of acquiring the infection to find out if it protects them from developing the disease. Some phase II trials may be controlled and randomized, with half the volunteers randomly allocated the drug or vaccine while the other (control) half are given a placebo—a harmless, ineffective, but similarly packaged and delivered product. Also, the trial may be 'open-label' or 'blinded'; the former meaning that the investigators and participants know who gets which formulation whereas in the latter case participants are not given this information until the trial is over. If statistical analysis of trial results determines that the product is safe and effective, then a large, phase III trial is launched, which is double-blind (meaning that neither participants nor investigators know who gets the test or control product), and placebo-controlled. As with phase II trials, this would involve those with the disease when investigating a new drug or those at high risk of developing the disease if investigating a vaccine. These trials are again testing for efficacy and safety and often recruit several thousand participants. The exact number required is calculated to give a statistically significant result, which clearly indicates whether the drug or vaccine is either effective or ineffective against the microbe in question. With statistically significant results from a phase III trial, the final step is to submit the data to the licensing authorities (the Food and Drug Administration (FDA) in the US and the Medicines and Healthcare Products Regulatory Agency in the UK) so that the product can be approved for clinical use.

Since this series of clinical trials takes so long to complete, the 2014–16 Ebola epidemic would probably have been over before they were completed and any effective drug or vaccine could be licensed for general use. What's more, the traditional method of testing involves thousands of participants but denies half of them any benefits that the candidate drug or vaccine might afford. So from an ethical standpoint some regard this as unacceptable during an epidemic of a disease with mortality rates as high as those of Ebola. As we will see, these ethical issues caused much debate among those responsible for designing and running trials of potential Ebola vaccines and drugs during the epidemic.

*   *   *

At the start of the Ebola epidemic in 2014, supportive treatment was all that could be offered to most Ebola sufferers in West Africa. This support is detailed in the 'Guidelines for caring for patients with filovirus haemorrhagic fevers' (caused by Ebola and Marburg viruses) published by MSF[1] and includes providing drugs to relieve common, distressing Ebola symptoms such as fever, pain, nausea, vomiting, anxiety, and confusion. The guidelines also stress the importance of nutritional support for patients, indicating that food should be 'easy to digest, well balanced and culturally acceptable', and that 'families should also be allowed to provide food for their relatives, as this food is likely to be more acceptable by the patients'. Because of the similarity between early stage Ebola symptoms and those of several other, common infections, MSF also recommend that all patients admitted to treatment centres receive anti-malarial drugs and a broad spectrum antibiotic for potential concurrent, undiagnosed, tropical diseases. But, as discussed earlier, the mainstay of Ebola patient care is fluid balance—that is balancing fluid input with output— to prevent the complications of severe dehydration.

In the early stages of Ebola, adequate rehydration can generally be achieved by encouraging patients to drink an oral rehydration solution, but if/when severe vomiting and/or diarrhoea occur intravenous fluid replacement is required. At this stage it is important to correct electrolyte/metabolic disturbances; in particular potassium levels, which are often low, a state that can cause sudden death from cardiac arrhythmias. Yet the problems involved in monitoring and correcting electrolyte balance in an Ebola isolation ward with limited laboratory backup in West Africa are immense. Even inserting intravenous infusion lines puts health care workers at risk of infection, and the constant blood monitoring and delicate adjustments required to maintain electrolyte balance pose additional risks to isolation ward and laboratory workers. A report from an Ebola treatment centre in Conakry, Guinea, early in the epidemic, stresses the difficulties encountered: '[T]here were approximately three clinical rounds per day, with two or three doctors and two or three nurses for each round, and depending on the type of personal protective equipment that was used, rounds were limited to either 1 hour or 3 hours because of the intense heat and humidity inside some types of personal protective equipment. Although we attempted to deliver oral and intravenous fluids to correct dehydration and metabolic abnormalities, care was still suboptimal. With more clinical personnel in each treatment center, better supportive care could be delivered more consistently, and we think that mortality could be driven lower.' Nevertheless, the mortality rate reported in this study was 43%,[2] well below the overall ~66% rate for the whole country at the time.

Unsurprisingly, the few Ebola sufferers repatriated to hospitals in Westernized countries (such as Ian Crozier mentioned earlier) received more intensive therapy than those in treatment centres in West Africa. Virtually all were offered experimental drugs and several were given infusions of convalescent plasma, but most important was access to sophisticated fluid and electrolyte balance. In the case of an American doctor who contracted Ebola in Liberia and was repatriated to Emory University Hospital, Atlanta, up to five litres of intravenous fluid a day were required for seven days in addition to his oral fluid intake to compensate for diarrhoeal fluid loss.[3] During this time the patient's heart rate was constantly monitored and when cardiac irregularities occurred they were immediately treated by the addition of more potassium chloride to the infusion. Although no formal clinical trials have been conducted to assess the benefit of fluid replacement to Ebola survival, comparisons between Ebola sufferers admitted to treatment centres who received adequate fluid replacement and those who remained in the community without such treatment, show at least 10% increased survival in the former group.

*   *   *

In August 2014, WHO convened the first of a series of meetings of experts to review potential Ebola treatments, to prioritize the most promising and fast track their progress through phase I trials. Ethical committees and licensing authorities also acted with unprecedented speed in a bid to complete phase I trials in non-epidemic regions and begin phase II and III trials in West Africa while there were sufficient Ebola cases to provide meaningful results.

One treatment prioritized by WHO was the infusion of convalescent plasma donated by Ebola survivors. This was the earliest type of specific treatment developed for Ebola, first pioneered during the Ebola outbreak in Yambuku in 1976. The aim is simple; to provide passive immunity, in the form of Ebola-specific antibodies, to an Ebola sufferer to help their immune system fight the virus. Although stocks were limited, Ebola convalescent plasma has been used to treat a handful of patients in several outbreaks since 1976, but no clinical trials were conducted and so any benefit that this treatment might bestow was still unproven in 2014. Yet, even if Ebola convalescent plasma did prove efficacious, it is obviously not the most convenient type of treatment as it requires expensive, sophisticated plasmapheresis equipment to prepare the plasma and it could prove difficult to generate enough stocks for use on the scale required for a large epidemic.

Because of these constraints, a study that began in Sierra Leone in late 2014 tested the benefit of infusing compatible whole blood rather than plasma taken from the increasing numbers of Ebola survivors who were keen to help other sufferers. Survivors' blood contains the required Ebola-specific antibodies and is much easier to obtain than purified plasma. Initial results comparing disease outcome in infused and non-infused patients looked promising with thirty-three of forty-four treated patients (75%) surviving.[4] But by February 2015 plasmapheresis machines had been imported into West Africa and a non-randomized, comparative trial began at the Ebola treatment centre run by MSF in Conakry, Guinea. Two doses of 250ml of convalescent plasma from different donors were given to consenting adults within two days of receiving a laboratory diagnosis of Ebola. The primary outcome measured was the risk of death between three and sixteen days after diagnosis. Results from eighty-four infused patients were compared with 418 patients who received only supportive treatment at the same treatment centre over the previous five months. The risk of death was 31% in the convalescent plasma group and 38% in the control group, a difference that was not statistically significant. So the authors of the published report concluded that 'The transfusion of

up to 500ml of convalescent plasma…in 84 patients with confirmed EVD [Ebola virus disease] was not associated with significant improvement in survival.'[5] However, they stressed that they
were not able to measure levels of virus neutralizing antibody in
the infusions because they had no access to a bio-safety level 4 laboratory, and suggested that these levels may be an important factor in determining whether an infusion will be beneficial or not.

While the whole procedure of collecting and testing convalescent plasma from Ebola survivors for therapeutic use is somewhat
cumbersome, time-consuming, and expensive, purified, specific
antibodies generated in the laboratory, called *monoclonal antibodies*,
can be produced at reasonable cost and in unlimited amounts.
Prior to 2014 three such antibodies existed that were known
to inhibit Ebola virus replication in the test tube. These three antibodies were combined into a biopharmaceutical antibody cocktail
called ZMapp, which was produced commercially by genetically
manipulated tobacco plants that contained the antibody-coding
genes by a technique called 'pharming'.[6] A report that appeared in
2014,[7] described the results of testing ZMapp efficacy in Ebola-
infected rhesus monkeys (*Macaca mulatta*), and showed that ZMapp
protected 100% of infected monkeys against lethal Ebola while all
control, infected but untreated monkeys died of the disease.
Importantly, the antibody cocktail was also effective when administered up to five days after the animals were infected with
the virus—an incredibly encouraging result. ZMapp immediately
became the front-runner for effective, post-exposure Ebola
treatment.

Publication of this report caused quite a stir. Everyone knew
that demonstrating efficacy of a product in a relevant animal
model was just the first step to getting it licensed for use in

humans, but with a lethal epidemic raging in West Africa, most felt that any agent with possible beneficial effects should be made available to Ebola sufferers as soon as possible. Indeed, a report from WHO's panel of experts stated that 'the panel reached a consensus that it is ethical to offer unproven interventions [for Ebola] with as yet unknown efficacy and adverse effects, as potential treatment or prevention.'[8] Perhaps this *is* a reasonable approach under the exceptional circumstances, but other experts warned that 'this is an inferior strategy and that instead, RCT [randomized controlled trials] should be used from the early stages of human experimentation of candidate Ebola interventions.'[9]

In an unprecedented act, the FDA allowed ZMapp to be used for Ebola treatment in American patients. But this decision caused further controversy between those who called for this and other experimental products to be made available in West Africa as soon as phase I safety trials were completed and others who had reservations about such a strategy. In the former camp were three eminent scientists with many years' experience of fighting epidemics in resource-poor countries. In an article in the *Wall Street Journal*,[10] Jeremy Farrar (Director of the Wellcome Trust), David Heymann (Head of Chatham House Centre on Global Security), and Peter Piot (Director of the London School of Hygiene and Tropical Medicine) argued strongly that, in the unlikely event of Ebola spreading in the West, patients and those at risk of infection would certainly be offered experimental drugs and vaccines on a compassionate basis. Indeed, they cite the case of a German virologist who in 2001 accidently pricked her finger with the needle of a syringe containing *Zaire Ebola virus*. As there was no drug or vaccine even in clinical trials at the time, she was offered an experimental vaccine that had shown some protective properties in primates but had never been tested in humans. Faced with the possibility of developing a deadly disease, she accepted the vaccine as the best option available. She did not develop Ebola, but of course she may never have been infected with the virus in the first place. Be that as it may, the point is that she was offered a non-licensed, experimental product. These three scientists felt strongly that the same opportunity should be given to those with, or at risk of catching, Ebola in West Africa.

Those opposed to this view stressed the sensitivities involved in using Western-style medicines in West Africa, fearing the outcome if experimental treatments either proved ineffective or caused harm. With all the mistrust of Western medicine already witnessed in the early stages of the epidemic, the US authorities would at least be severely criticized for using Africans as guinea pigs for American drug companies and, worse, be accused of actually causing the epidemic with their drugs. While Farrar, Heymann, and Piot were familiar with these risks, they argued that 'African governments should be allowed to make informed decisions about whether or not to use these products, for example to protect and treat health-care workers who run especially high risk of infection.' They added, 'the West must fast-track safety testing of drugs and vaccines in unaffected countries, so that those which perform well could go into fuller trials in the affected region before the outbreak ends.' They urged WHO to take a leadership role in assisting the worst affected African countries in developing protocols for using and testing these treatment and prevention options.

WHO *did* prioritize ZMapp for trials in West Africa but despite all the rush there was a disappointing end for this promising product. In the US, just seven Ebola sufferers were treated with it, two of whom died. No conclusions regarding its efficacy could be drawn from this small, uncontrolled group. A ZMapp clinical trial was planned in Liberia by a research partnership between the Liberian Ministry of Health and the US National Institutes of Health, but stocks were low and took a while to be replenished. The trial that finally began in March 2015 was fraught with difficulties from the start. With patient numbers diminishing by the day, recruitment was extended to include cases in Sierra Leone and Guinea and it finally enrolled around 72 cases.[11] All participants received optimized standard care and half were randomized also to receive three injections of ZMapp. When numbers of deaths at twenty-eight days were compared between the two groups, the results showed 37% deaths in the control group and 22% in the ZMapp group, a difference that is not statistically significant.[12]

One anti-viral drug, favipiravir (also called T-705) was already in clinical use in 2014 and was considered for trials against Ebola. It had completed phase I and II trials successfully and was licensed for use against the 'flu virus in Japan where it is manufactured by Fujifilm RI Pharma. Rapid testing in 2014 showed that the drug had anti-Ebola activity both in the test tube and in laboratory mice.[13]

In December 2014 the JIKI clinical trial, described as a phase II, multi-centre, non-controlled trial, began in Guinea with the remit to test the efficacy of favipiravir in reducing mortality in individuals infected by Ebola virus. The trial was conducted in collaboration with MSF and other NGOs in four Ebola treatment centres. Consenting adults and children over one year of age received the drug for ten days along with basic care and their fatality rate was compared with controls treated at the same centres before the trial began. After treating just eighty patients the researchers presented preliminary results that they judged 'should be quickly shared with the international community'. The overall fatality rates were 48% for treated patients and 58% for historical controls; not a statistically significant result. Notably though, the fatality rate among Ebola sufferers who received the drug in the early stages of the disease when their viral loads were low was 15% and this compared favourably with the control group in which the death rate was 30%. However, favipiravir had no influence on the fatality rate (85%) among Ebola patients who arrived at treatment centres in the late stages of the disease and with high viral loads.[14]

Following this announcement all Ebola patients in Guinea received favipiravir. But if assessing efficacy was the intended outcome, then there was a basic flaw in the trial design—it was not randomized or effectively controlled. The drug was given to all participants and the outcome compared with that of historical Ebola cases. Clearly, the reason for this was humanitarian but, inevitably, scientists not involved in the trial were sceptical about the results. Their view was that Ebola survival critically depends on the quality of care received, and this may have been subtly different for the historical cases, so influencing the results. Additionally, the drug was only beneficial in cases who were more likely to survive Ebola even without specific treatment.

Several other drug trials began in West Africa during 2015 but, for one reason or another, did not come to fruition. A case in point was a drug called TKM-Ebola-Guinea, which had been used to treat two American Ebola sufferers (one was Ian Crozier), both of whom survived. There were high hopes for this drug as it had been specifically constructed by Tekmira Pharmaceuticals in Canada to interfere with replication of the Makona strain of Ebola virus. Studies were fast-tracked by WHO and FDA after TKM-Ebola-Guinea showed promising results against Ebola in monkeys. An interesting trial design was adopted whereby on days when trial enrolment capacity was reached, all following patients were enrolled into an observational (control) cohort.[15] But after treating just fourteen Ebola patients with the drug in Sierra Leone the trial was terminated by the company, which stated that the drug did not seem to be effective.

One intriguing result came from a chance event in the treatment centre run by MSF in Foya, Liberia, at the height of the epidemic. In accordance with MSF guidelines, all patients admitted to the centre were routinely given the anti-malarial drug combination artemether-lumefantrine on admission. But for a twelve-day period in August 2014 when the centre was admitting over 100 new Ebola cases a week, the supply of this drug combination ran out and was replaced with an alternative combination—artesunate-amodiaquine—while all other treatment remained unchanged. Because amodiaquine had previously been found to have some anti-Ebola activity in the test tube, scientists compared the disease outcome between patients receiving the two drug combinations and found a 31% lower risk of death in the artesunate -amodiaquine group[16]—clearly a finding that requires further investigation.

* * *

Overall the hope that the 2014–16 Ebola epidemic would act as a testing ground for Ebola-specific drugs failed to materialize. The major problem was that no potentially useful product was ready and waiting when the epidemic first hit. Consequently, most trials only began after the epidemic had peaked and inevitably several failed to enrol sufficient patients to produce clearcut results. In fact, with diminishing patient numbers, trials seemed to be competing with each other for patients, thereby preventing any one from delivering meaningful results. So while at the start of the epidemic WHO was severely criticized for doing *too little too late*, with the trials they supported it was *too many too late*. In addition, most trials lacked a control arm and therefore gave inconclusive results. While it is understandable on humanitarian grounds to give an experimental treatment to all sufferers, many scientists think that WHO officials should have been more insistent on a randomized, controlled design for all trials or been more open to alternative trial designs. Only then would we be in a better position to save lives in the next Ebola outbreak.

Sadly, a unique opportunity was lost, but thankfully, with the benefit of some creative designs, Ebola vaccine trials fared rather better than the drug trials. When a WHO team of experts met in September 2014 to discuss potential Ebola vaccine trials there were two front-runners, both of which had shown 100% efficacy in preventing Ebola virus disease in infected, non-human primates[17] and were just entering phase I trials in humans. One of these was developed at the US National Institutes of Health in collaboration with the pharmaceutical company GlaxoSmithKline. The vaccine, called cAD3-EBO, used an inactivated chimpanzee adenovirus, genetically engineered to express the gene for Ebola glycoprotein, as a vehicle for delivering this protein to vaccinees so that they mounted an immune response against it. Ebola glycoprotein is found in the outer coat of *Zaire Ebola virus*, and induces a protective immune response during natural infection by blocking virus entry into host cells. In phase I trials conducted in the US in September 2014, twenty volunteers were given a single shot of either a low or a high dose of the vaccine. All developed an immune response against Ebola glycoprotein, but those who received the high dose produced higher levels of antibodies and also generated Ebola-specific immune T cells, cells that have been shown to correlate with protective immunity in non-human primates.[18]

The second front-runner Ebola vaccine was under development by the Public Health Agency of Canada in association with the pharmaceutical company Merck. This vaccine, rVSV, uses live vesicular stomatitis virus genetically engineered to express the same *Zaire Ebola virus* glycoprotein. Vesicular stomatitis virus naturally infects cattle, horses, deer, and pigs, causing blisters and ulcers in the mouth as well as on the tongue, feet, and teats. The disease is mild and infected animals recover within a week or so. The virus can also jump from livestock to humans, when it is either asymptomatic or causes a mild 'flu-like illness.

Live (as opposed to inactivated) virus vaccines are used because the virus actually infects and grows in vaccinees, expressing high levels of the foreign protein (in this case Ebola glycoprotein) over a long period of time. This generally induces a rapid, strong, protective immune response which may be more enduring than that produced by an inactivated vaccine. However, live vaccines usually cause more adverse reactions than their inactivated counterparts and so extensive phase I trials of rVSV were undertaken to check on both its safety and immunogenicity. In fact, three open-label, dose-escalation trials and one randomized, double-blind, controlled, phase I trial were completed, enrolling a total of 158 healthy adults in Europe and Africa. Although no vaccinee experienced a serious adverse reaction, several transient symptoms classified as mild-to-moderate were reported, including fever and arthritis in up to 35% and 22% of vaccinees respectively. While these adverse effects were more common in groups receiving higher doses of vaccine, all doses induced an Ebola-specific immune response after a single vaccine shot, so a dose that was effective and caused acceptable adverse reactions could be selected.[19]

In February 2015 the Partnership for Research on Ebola Vaccines in Liberia (PREVAIL) clinical trial opened. It was described as a phase II/III trial designed to evaluate the safety and efficacy of the cAD3 and rVSV vaccines.[20] While PREVAIL conformed to the classic randomized, double-blind, controlled trial design, it was a three-arm trial, with two vaccine arms being compared with one control arm, and so the majority (two-thirds) of volunteers received a vaccine that might protect against Ebola while just one third receive a placebo. The trial, led by a Liberia–US partnership and sponsored by the US National Institutes of Health, aimed to enrol 27,000 healthy men and women over 18 years of age in ten vaccination centres in and around Monrovia. Women who were either pregnant or breast feeding were excluded from the trial because of potential adverse reactions from the live virus in the rVSV vaccine, while those at high risk of Ebola, such as health care workers, burial team members, and ambulance drivers were actively sought out for enrolment.

In September 2014, while this large trial was being planned, CDC scientists devised a mathematical model which predicted that 'without additional interventions or changes in community behaviour (eg notable reductions in unsafe burial practices), the model also estimates that Liberia and Sierra Leone will have approximately 550,000 Ebola cases (1.4 million when corrected for under reporting).'[21] With these huge predictions, PREVAIL organizers must have expected not only to trial the two vaccines successfully but also to protect thousands of people from Ebola infection. But it was not to be. As we now know, by the end of January 2015 the peak of the epidemic had passed and from then on Ebola case numbers fell continuously. Extremely welcome as this turn of events was to all concerned, it clearly threatened the power of the trial by decreasing the likelihood of sufficient Ebola cases occurring in its test and control arms. In the event PREVAIL was downgraded to a phase II study after enrolling just 1,500 participants. At this point two more trials were started using single-shot rVSV, one in Sierra Leone and the other in Guinea, targeting high-risk populations and with a rather less conventional design.

The first of these was STRIVE (Sierra Leone Trial to Introduce a Vaccine against Ebola) sponsored by CDC.[22] This trial selected chiefdoms within the five Sierra Leonean districts hardest hit by Ebola and targeted all staff within selected health care facilities. The study was un-blinded and individually randomized, with no placebo. Once enrolled, participants were randomly assigned for either immediate vaccination within seven days or deferred vaccination eighteen to twenty-four weeks later. All participants were followed up for six months after vaccination for development of Ebola virus disease, vaccine safety checks and a subset was tested for level and duration of the Ebola-specific immune response—a crucial parameter in understanding the vaccine's potential for inducing long-term protection. The deferred group acted as a non-vaccinated group for comparison until they in turn were vaccinated. This study began in April 2015, at which time around four Ebola cases per week were being reported in Sierra Leone. To date STRIVE has enrolled over 8,650 participants but at the time of writing no data on the trial have been released. It seems unlikely that there will be sufficient Ebola cases among participants to give statistically significant results, but nevertheless, the trial will provide important data on vaccine safety and the immune responses it generates.

The second unconventional trial using the rVSV vaccine was called Ebola ça Suffit (Ebola this is enough).[23] This had an open-label, cluster-randomized, ring vaccination design and was organized by WHO. It began in April 2015 in Basse-Guinea, a coastal area of Guinea including Conakry and eight other prefectures. The ring vaccination approach was first used during the smallpox eradication campaign in the 1970s and is defined as: 'the vaccination of a cluster of individuals at high risk of infection owing to their social or geographical connection to a confirmed index case'.[24] In Ebola ça Suffit the index case was a newly diagnosed case of Ebola and the cluster included all the contacts and contacts-of-contacts of this case. Contacts were defined as: individuals who, within the last twenty-one days, lived in the same household, were visited by the index case after the onset of symptoms, or were in close physical contact with the patient's body or bodily fluids, linen, or clothes. Contacts-of-contacts included neighbours, family, or extended family members living within the nearest geographical boundary of all contacts, plus household members of any high-risk contacts.

Each cluster was randomly assigned to have immediate or delayed vaccination and consenting adults, excluding Ebola survivors and pregnant and lactating women, were either vaccinated directly or twenty-one days later. The primary outcome measure was laboratory confirmed Ebola virus disease with onset at least ten days after randomization. This ten-day period was set to exclude cases occurring in those who were already infected before vaccination and to cover for the unknown time it takes for the vaccine to induce protective immunity.

In August 2015 the team published interim results of the trial up to July 20, 2015, by which time ninety clusters had been randomized. This included a total of 7,651 participants with forty-eight clusters getting the vaccine immediately and forty-two receiving it twenty-one days later. Comparison of the incidence of Ebola in all vaccinated individuals in the immediate vaccination group with all those in the delayed vaccination group showed that at ten days or more after randomization there had been zero cases in the immediate group and sixteen in the delayed group. This gives an estimated vaccine efficacy of 100% and statistical calculations reveal a 95% chance that the vaccine's efficacy is between 75 and 100%.[25] This publication was greeted with unanimous enthusiasm and applause—at last, a product that works against Ebola!

With such convincing data, at the end of July 2015 the Ebola ça Suffit trial stopped randomizing and all contacts were offered the vaccine immediately. In addition, at the time of writing the vaccine is being used to vaccinate the contacts of every new case of Ebola in Guinea, Sierra Leone, and Liberia.

With this success in the bag, more detailed studies are ongoing to prepare for the next Ebola outbreak. In particular, for each vaccine preparation it is important to assess how quickly immunity develops after vaccination and how long it lasts. Only then will we know which vaccine to use in particular situations. In this regard, during the Ebola ça Suffit trial Ebola cases *did* in fact occur in the immediate vaccination arm, but as they developed within ten days of vaccination they were assumed to have been due to an infection prior to vaccination and were therefore excluded from the analysis. These cases highlight the importance of knowing how long it takes to develop protective immunity after vaccination as well as whether a vaccine can provide post exposure prevention. The answers to these key questions will vary according to vaccine preparations and vaccination schedules. It is likely that more than one vaccine will be required to cover all eventualities, including rapid development of immunity for case contacts and long-term immunity for health care workers and the general population.

With these variables in mind, other phase II vaccine trials are in the pipeline, one of which, called EBOVAC–Salone (run by the London School of Hygiene and Tropical Medicine, Jensen Pharmaceutical Companies of Johnson and Johnson, and Sierra Leone's Ministry of Health and Sanitation), was launched in Kambia District, Sierra Leone, in early 2016. This uses two Ebola glycoprotein-based vaccines in a prime-boost strategy, meaning that participants first get a priming dose of an adenovirus vaccine (AD26. ZEBOV) to stimulate the immune system followed two months later by a boosting dose of modified vaccinia Ankara virus (MVA-BN-filo) to increase the Ebola-specific immune response. MVA is a virus that is unable to replicate in humans and has been widely used in vaccines against smallpox. This protocol gave no adverse reactions in phase I trials and now the team are enrolling healthy volunteers, including children, the elderly, and people living with HIV, with the intent of studying the fine details of the immune response to the vaccine.[26]

Hopefully, this prime-boost approach will produce long-term protection against Ebola and this and other vaccine trials will leave us much better prepared for the next Ebola epidemic than we were in 2014. But we are still without drugs with a proven beneficial effect on the Ebola virus disease.

9

~

Lessons Learned

After a two-year battle against Ebola, the epidemic in West Africa was finally declared over in January 2016. By then the virus had infected over 28,000 people and killed more than 11,000 of them. Never before has an Ebola outbreak killed so many, transcended national borders, or lasted so long. This was the time for some in-depth analysis of the response to the crisis and for laying plans to ensure that such a humanitarian calamity never happens again.

Many linked factors combined to allow the initial Ebola outbreak in Guinea to evolve into an epidemic of unprecedented proportions. Principally, the lack of Ebola expertise in West Africa resulted in early failure to implement the WHO guidelines for controlling Ebola outbreaks, so allowing the virus to get a head start. This was compounded by inadequate health infrastructure, delayed identification of the disease, downplaying the full extent of the outbreak by national authorities, WHO's failure to recognize the severity of the problem, poor coordination of epidemic management between Guinea, Sierra Leone, and Liberia, and local mistrust in government authorities and Western medicine.

Two events finally persuaded WHO and international governments to sit up and take notice—repatriation of two US aid workers suffering from Ebola, and the virus's jump from Liberia to Nigeria. Both incidents caught world media attention, and although Nigeria only suffered a minor outbreak, with twenty cases and eight deaths, it acted as a global wake-up call. If Ebola could fly to Nigeria unheeded then nowhere was safe—not even the leafy suburbs of rich Westernized cities. Suddenly WHO and international governments were engaged and the fight back began in earnest.

With case numbers growing exponentially between August and December 2014, curbing the epidemic critically depended on a workforce of volunteers and army recruits joining with international agencies and local community members to stop virus spread. Once up and running, the scale and vitality of the international response was truly extraordinary. The UK, committed to supporting the Sierra Leonean Government, funded treatment centres, Ebola testing laboratories, and community care centres. British army personnel undertook construction work, set up training programmes, and organized burial teams. Over 150 UK National Health Service, PHE, and university staff volunteered for frontline service in treatment centres and another 100 or so volunteers staffed the Ebola testing laboratories. Overall the UK delivered 2,800,000 kilos of supplies, including one million personal protective suits and 200 vehicles.[1] A remarkable list; but the UK did not act alone. The US and France masterminded the response in Liberia and Guinea respectively while the African Union, the Economic Community of West Africa, China, Canada, Cuba, and many other countries contributed personnel, funding, logistics, and technology, and private companies and foundations supplied funds and in-kind assistance. But most impressive were the thousands of individuals, both national and international, who risked their lives to care for Ebola patients, collect and test blood samples, seek out and monitor potential cases, drive ambulances, transport laboratory specimens, bury the dead, wash contaminated laundry, and scrub boots. The list of brave workers goes on and on; without them this war against Ebola could not have been won.

Nevertheless, mistakes were made and inadequacies exposed. WHO is responsible for warning the world of potential epidemics through its Global Alert and Response Programme (incidentally, set up after the Kikwit Ebola outbreak in 1995). It also has a remit to respond appropriately to outbreak situations. In this regard, WHO's performance during the 2014–16 epidemic was severely criticized. International governments, NGOs, and groups of experts pointed the finger at WHO not only for the delay in sounding the alarm but also for its poorly functioning regional and country offices and a lack of leadership and coordination on the ground in West Africa.

So what exactly is required to ensure that the world is protected from, and can respond to, Ebola and other potential pandemic infections in future? In the aftermath of Ebola several experts proposed answers to this question, including an independent panel lead by Harvard Global Health Institute, and the London School of Hygiene and Tropical Medicine, which published a wide-ranging report in November 2015 entitled 'Will Ebola Change the Game? Ten Essential Reforms Before the Next Pandemic'.[2] Their recommendations for global health security included: 1) setting up and providing governance for global monitoring systems that will predict major outbreaks; 2) responding to infectious disease outbreaks in a sufficient and timely manner; and 3) researching the cause, treatment, and prevention of major disease outbreaks. Depressingly, these recommendations look very like those published after other outbreaks including Ebola in Kikwit in 1995. We know what has to be done; the question is: has the death toll and suffering of the 2014–16 Ebola epidemic motivated international decision-making bodies and funders sufficiently for them to bite the bullet this time round?

*　*　*

WHO admitted its failures during the early stages of the Ebola epidemic and in response set up an Advisory Group on WHO's Work in Outbreak and Emergencies which presented its final report to the Director General in January 2016. The group proposed a new WHO Programme on Outbreaks and Emergencies with a defined budget, a single workforce that would answer directly to the Director General and have the flexibility and adaptability to deal with the multi-faceted nature of health and humanitarian emergencies robustly and quickly, assessing the risks, raising the alarm and taking a leadership role in the response on the ground.[3] This all sounds encouraging but the new programme will only be as good as its funding allows. In recent years WHO has suffered financial cuts with consequent loss of staff from many programmes. While efficiency savings can go so far, the Organization relies on its 194 member states for its budget. But despite all member states endorsing universal health coverage as a guiding principle, each year several states, including some rich Western nations, do not pay up. At the World Health Assembly in 2015, Director General Margaret Chan asked member states to increase their contributions by just 5%; they refused. As Chan said: 'If you want WHO to be strong and fit for purpose, keep your promises. Put your money where your mouth is. But many governments support a zero nominal-growth policy [for their contributions]. Maintaining that policy for 10 years has reduced the purchasing power of my budget by about one-third.'[4]

Member states that refuse to pay their dues justify their action by accusing WHO of not being fit for purpose. Clearly, a well-functioning WHO with a reliable funding stream derived from fair contributions by all member states is essential if it is to provide world health security in the twenty-first century. Hopefully, the 2014–16 Ebola epidemic will stimulate the changes required to put this in place.

A global system for preventing and responding to outbreaks needs strong leadership and robust measures of accountability. To this end the Independent Panel of Experts recommended the creation of a Global Health Committee as part of the UN Security Council 'to expedite high-level leadership and systematically elevate political attention to health issues, recognising health as essential to human security.'[5] They also thought it imperative for WHO to rebuild trust by implementing governance reforms and focusing on its core functions. With an eye on 2017, when Chan steps down and there will be a change at the top of WHO, and in what appears to be a thinly veiled criticism of her leadership, the panel recommended that 'member states should insist on a Director-General with the character and capacity to challenge even the most powerful governments when necessary to protect public health.'[6]

*   *   *

Infectious disease microbes recognize no state or country boundaries, so in today's 'global village' an outbreak anywhere is a potential threat everywhere. All governments must invest in adequate, country-wide disease surveillance and early reporting systems which feed information from the grass roots to WHO's Outbreak and Emergencies Programme. In reality, to succeed this will require economic incentives for early reporting, and assurances from WHO that reporting will not result in trade and travel restrictions without justification (a fear that led governments to downplay the extent of the Ebola outbreak in 2014). WHO estimates that at least twenty-eight countries, which included Guinea, Sierra Leone, and Liberia even before 2014, do not have adequate health care systems, and without these in place surveillance systems cannot function. The world will always be at risk of future outbreaks until these services improve. So building capacity in poorer countries, where, at present, most potential pandemics begin, is essential and will necessitate external financial and technical support. While in the aftermath of the Ebola epidemic the World Bank and rich nations pledged funds to rebuild primary health care systems in the three worst affected countries (estimated at a cost of $2.1 billion), it is questionable whether funds will be forthcoming to help other poor nations to reach the required health care standards in the near future.

*   *   *

With respect to Ebola in particular, knowledge that the virus can persist in the body of survivors for many months after recovery and spread to others via sexual transmission, is a cause for grave concern. It is probable that, following the recent, or perhaps the next, epidemic, Ebola will maintain a chain of infection in humans and become endemic in remote areas of Africa where single cases or small, family outbreaks may go unnoticed or undiagnosed. For this reason alone it is essential that adequate surveillance systems are urgently established in West Africa so that Ebola can be recognized and dealt with at an early stage.

To this end, WHO, CDC, and international governments are working with in-country teams to rebuild primary care capacity which disappeared during the epidemic and also implementing disease surveillance and early reporting systems. For instance, in Sierra Leone, Public Health England, WHO, CDC, and the Sierra Leonean Ministry of Health formed an 'Ebola Transition Group' as early as May 2015. The aim was to harness the capacity built up during the epidemic and ensure that responsibility, accountability, and skills required for an effective, country-wide public health system were transferred from the National Ebola Response Centre, run predominantly by an international team, back to the Sierra Leonean Ministry of Health and Sanitation and Office of National Security. So when the epidemic ended in January 2016, there was already an Operational Response Centre within the Ministry ready to resume responsibility for public health surveillance. But there is still much to be done in building long-term capacity in the country before the whole system is fit for purpose. The aim is to have a National Reference Laboratory in Freetown at the hub of a network of four regional and several hospital-based laboratories by 2018.

Equipment from the laboratories hastily built for Ebola testing during the epidemic is being relocated to newly refurbished regional facilities, the first of which was up and running in Makeni by November 2015. These laboratories will be used to train a cadre of local laboratory workers to replace those who died of Ebola and to provide continuity. In the longer term an Institute for Sanitation, Water and Public Health is planned for Freetown to provide training in every aspect of public health.

Stimulated by the Ebola epidemic, great technological advances have been made in Ebola diagnostic testing. Rapid, accurate,

PCR-based, Ebola diagnostic test kits were developed, and field validation studies carried out, while the epidemic was still ongoing.[7] Now, finger-stick, point-of-care Ebola testing can be performed in minutes. So blood samples tested locally can then be forwarded to regional laboratories where, if negative for Ebola, will be tested for up to forty-five common, and not so common, infections including Lassa fever, dengue fever, yellow fever, Rift valley fever, chikungunya, and Ebola and Marburg viruses, all in one rapid, multiplex PCR-based test.

*   *   *

The 2014–16 Ebola epidemic may be over, yet the virus remains hidden in an animal reservoir, poised to strike again. Frustratingly, despite huge efforts during the epidemic, we are no nearer identifying the culprit animal species involved. While certain species of fruit bat are the prime suspects, the evidence is still weak, and fruit bat testing in West Africa during the epidemic drew a complete blank. In fact, after the search in Guinea in 2014 the finger was pointed at insect-eating bats, although this link is still only circumstantial.

Uncovering the animal reservoir of Ebola is essential to identify communities at risk and perhaps even prevent the virus striking again. Teams of animal hunters are planning surveys of West African species, but again money is the problem. The scientists are just hoping that with the memory of the Ebola epidemic still fresh in the mind, funding for field trips will be forthcoming. Most agree that the reservoir (or *reservoirs*, as there may be more than one species involved) is likely to be in a species that is hunted for food, but while some scientists are convinced that bats are the culprit, others disagree and call for a wide-ranging search including rodents, livestock, domestic dogs, cats, arthropods, and even fungi.[8] Wherever the virus is hiding, we must find it. Only then can we devise precautions against it jumping to humans again; these might include education and publicity campaigns, warnings, or bans on consumption.

*   *   *

The 2014–16 Ebola epidemic uncovered a major problem with research and development of drugs and vaccines for rare, epidemic diseases. Indeed, the fact that there were *any* anti-Ebola agents in the pipeline in 2014 was entirely because of its perceived bioterrorist threat in the West. In the event, patients were left with no specific treatment or prevention options, resulting in unacceptably high levels of suffering and death while health care workers put their lives at risk in endeavouring to care for the sick and eradicate the virus. Everyone agrees that such a situation should not be allowed to happen again, but how can we insure against it?

In truth, the global community faces a number of pandemic threats from natural, accidental, or purposeful release of an infectious agent. To be prepared for these outbreaks we need weapons, in this case specific vaccines and drugs. But many microbes with the potential to cause an epidemic, such as Marburg, Lassa fever, Rift valley fever, Crimean-Congo haemorrhagic fever, Hendra and Nipah, West Nile fever, Middle East respiratory syndrome, and hanta viruses, are among the so-called 'neglected infectious disease pathogens', for which, like Ebola, development of specifically targeted agents is not commercially viable. Nevertheless, in order to react immediately to an outbreak of any one of these viruses it is essential to have a stockpile of drugs and vaccines ready to test in the field on day one. So who is going to foot the bill?

Developing such an arsenal is the vision of Jeremy Farrar, Director of the Wellcome Trust, UK, who holds the purse strings of the world's largest medical research charity and who, in the face of the Ebola epidemic, immediately committed $15.2 million (£10 million) to fund the only vaccine trial that gave positive results. But the problem is bigger than any single organization can confront. Farrar compares global health security with the global security in readiness for fighting wars and terrorism. In reality, over the centuries microbes have killed many more people than have wars or terrorists, yet while every country in the world has an army and a stockpile of weapons ready to protect its people against wars, there is a reluctance to commit the necessary funds to protect against similar threats from pandemic microbes.

Accepting that the pharmaceutical industry alone will not fund the development of drugs and vaccines that are not financially viable, Farrar argues that governments, NGOs, industry, and philanthropists must come together to fund research and development of outbreak-related drugs, vaccines, diagnostics, and essential kit such as personal protective equipment. In this regard, Farrar points to the success of GAVI, the Global Alliance Vaccine Initiative. Established in 2000, this initiative brings together public and private sectors to provide equal access to vaccines for children living in the world's poorest countries; an enormously successful venture that has saved countless lives. Farrar's mission is to set up an equivalent international alliance to provide resources for research and development of non-commercially viable drugs and vaccines.[9] He points out that a vaccine costs $500–1,000 million (£350–700 million) to take all the way from bench to bedside; in contrast, because of the absence of vaccines the Ebola emergency cost well over $8 billion (£5.7 billion). But memories are short, so Farrar is determined to act while the horrors of Ebola remain fresh in the mind—'2016 must be a year of action', he says.

POSTSCRIPT

Within a month of the Ebola epidemic ending, WHO declared another Public Health Emergency of International Concern, this time in relation to global spread of Zika virus. This virus, first isolated from Rhesus monkeys in Uganda in 1947, spreads between humans via a mosquito vector. For several years scientists have been tracking the virus from its origins in Africa and Asia, island hopping across the Pacific Ocean to South America and reaching Brazil in May 2015.[1] Zika caused outbreaks of a mainly mild 'flu-like illness at each stopover, and, at the time of writing, there is a huge Zika epidemic in Brazil with spread to other Latin American and Caribbean countries. While a mild 'flu-like illness is no cause for alarm, probable links between Zika infection and the birth defect microcephaly as well as the neurological condition Guillain-Barré syndrome, is the reason for WHO's declaration. Confirmation of these links is urgent, since Zika has the capability to become endemic throughout its vector's range—the whole region from South America to the southern states of the US and also southern Europe.

Once again the world has been caught unprepared for the crisis that Zika may cause. But this time it is understandable. Global surveillance systems successfully tracked Zika's progress, but no one regarded the virus as a sufficient threat to warrant drug and vaccine production. But the result is the same—we are in a reactive, catch-up situation. While accepting that we will always find ourselves in this predicament when new emerging microbes, like HIV and SARS, jump from their animal source for the first time, surely we have learned lessons from the Ebola epidemic that are applicable to Zika:

First, react quickly—it is better to be criticized for overreacting than for leaving the situation unattended to too long.

Second, innovative techniques should be tried out. For example, it should be possible to cut vaccine production from years to months by using innovative approaches such as adaptable platforms.[2] Fortunately, Zika virus is closely related to dengue fever virus (both are Flaviviruses) for which a vaccine has recently been licensed for use in humans. So using the dengue virus vaccine backbone that has passed safety testing, and replacing the dengue fever virus sequence in it for Zika genome sequences, pre-clinical workup, and phase 1 clinical trials could be completed rapidly.

Third, the classical series of clinical trials that can take ten years to complete before a new product can be licensed is not always appropriate. In emergency situations innovative approaches that provide efficacy and safety data at the same time as protecting participants (such as that used in Ebola ça Suffit) should be considered.

Finally, remember—nasty surprises will continue to emerge—we must learn to expect the unexpected.

GLOSSARY

Acquired Immunodeficiency Syndrome (AIDS) the stage of human immunodeficiency virus infection characterized by recurrent opportunistic infections.

Antibody a molecule that circulates in blood and body fluids and that binds to a specific target molecule, often on an infectious organism, thereby preventing infection.

Bacterium a unicellular micro-organism in the domain Bacteria.

Cardiac arrhythmia an irregular heartbeat.

CD4 see Lymphocytes.

Cerebrospinal fluid clear, colourless fluid found in and around the brain and spinal cord.

Chlorine solution 0.05% solution of sodium hypochlorite used as a chemical hand wash.

Cytokine a soluble chemical messenger that regulates immune responses.

Cytokine storm a massive, inappropriate release of cytokines following over-stimulation of the immune system.

DNA (deoxyribonucleic acid) a self-replicating molecule that carries the genetic material of all organisms except RNA viruses.

Endemic found regularly in a particular geographic area or population.

Epidemic a large-scale temporary increase in a disease in a community or region.

Epidemiology the study of the incidence, distribution, and control of diseases.

Endothelial cells the type of cells that line the interior surface of blood vessels.

Flu see Influenza.

Genome the genetic material of an organism.

Guillain-Barré syndrome peripheral nerve damage causing muscle weakness (sometimes leading to paralysis) following an infectious disease.

Haemorrhagic fever an infectious fever characterized by bleeding.

Herd immunity Indirect protection of a whole community from an infectious disease to which the majority have been immunized.

Herpes viruses a family of DNA viruses including those causing cold sores, chickenpox, and shingles.

Immune-privileged site see Sanctuary sites.

Immuno-pathology tissue damage caused by the immune response.

Incubation period the period of time between infection and the onset of symptoms.

Influenza a generally mild respiratory disease caused by the ortho-myxovirus, influenza virus.

Index case the first case of an infectious disease in a population from which all other cases are derived.

Interferon a family of cytokines with anti-viral properties.

Jaundice yellow colouration of the skin and conjunctiva associated with liver disease.

Lymphocytes white blood cells with a variety of subsets that orchestrate the specific immune response eg helper (CD4) T cells and cytotoxic (CD8) T cells.

Macrophage a mobile immune cell found in tissues where it initiates an immune response by producing cytokines. Macrophages engulf and destroy foreign and dead material.

Magnetic Resonance Imaging (MRI) a type of scan that uses magnetic fields and radio waves to produce internal images of the body.

Meningoencephalitis inflammation of the brain meninges (outer membranes) and brain tissue often caused by a virus.

Microbe a general term used to cover all microscopic organisms including bacteria, viruses, archaea, and the unicellular fungi and parasites.

Monoclonal antibody mono-specific antibodies made from a culture of cloned antibody-producing lymphocytes. Used as reagents and in immunotherapy.

Microcephaly a congenital condition with an abnormally small head with incomplete brain development.

Outbreak a small, local increase in numbers of cases of a specific disease.

Pandemic   an epidemic involving more than one continent at the same time.

Pan-uveitis   inflammation of both the anterior and posterior chambers of the eye.

Petechiae   a rash of small red spots caused by bleeding into the skin.

Photophobia   pain to the eyes caused by exposure to light.

Plasma   a yellow fluid component of blood in which the red and white cells are suspended.

Plasmapheresis   the process of separation of whole blood into its fluid and cellular component parts.

Polymerase chain reaction (PCR)   a technique for amplifying a single DNA sequence thousands or millions of times.

Primary infection   the illness caused by an organism the first time it infects an individual.

Ribonucleic acid (RNA)   one of the two types of nucleic acid that exist in nature, the other being DNA. RNA forms the genetic material of some viruses.

Sanctuary sites/immune-privileged sites   regions or organs of the body that immune cells cannot penetrate.

Smallpox   a severe, acute virus infection caused by *Variola major* and characterized by skin pocks.

T lymphocytes   see Lymphocytes.

Uveitis   inflammation of the anterior chamber of the eye.

Vaccine   material derived from an infectious organism introduced into the body to generate a protective immune response without disease.

Vaccinee   an individual who has received a vaccine.

Venepuncture   insertion of a needle into a vein usually with the intent of withdrawing blood.

Virus   a small infectious agent in the form of a particle that can only replicate inside a living cell.

Yellow fever virus   a mosquito-transmitted *flavivirus* that causes yellow fever.

Zoonosis/Zoonotic infection   an infectious disease in humans acquired from an animal source.

NOTES

INTRODUCTION

1 Crawford, DH. *Viruses: A Very Short Introduction* P 44. Oxford University Press. 2011.

CHAPTER 1

1 Ebola Haemorrhagic Fever in Zaire, 1976; report of an international commission. In: Bull. WHO.56:271–93, 1978.
2 Piot, P. In: *No Time to Lose* P 38. WW Norton and Company. New York. London. 2012.
3 Piot, P. In: *No Time to Lose* P 35. WW Norton and Company. New York. London. 2012.
4 Piot, P. In: *No Time to Lose* Parts 1 and 2. WW Norton and Company. New York. London. 2012.
5 Piot, P. In: *No Time to Lose* P 47. WW Norton and Company. New York. London. 2012.
6 Piot, P. In: *No Time to Lose* P 48. WW Norton and Company. New York. London. 2012.
7 Ebola Haemorrhagic Fever in Zaire, 1976; report of an international commission. In: Bull. WHO.56:271–93, 1978.
8 Ebola Haemorrhagic Fever in Zaire, 1976; report of an international commission. In: Bull. WHO.56:271–93, 1978.
9 Ebola Haemorrhagic Fever in Zaire, 1976; report of an international commission. In: Bull. WHO.56:271–93, 1978.

CHAPTER 2

1 Piot, P. In: *No Time to Lose* P 3. WW Norton and Company. New York. London. 2012.
2 Piot, P. In: *No Time to Lose* WW Norton and Company. New York. London. 2012.
3 Martin, GA. Marburg Virus Disease. Postgraduate Medical Journal 49, 542–6. 1973.
4 Gear, JSS, Cassel, GA, Gear, AJ, Trappler, B, et al. Outbreak of Marburg Virus Disease in Johannesburg. *BMJ* 29 November, 489–93. 1975.

5 Johnson, KM, Lange, JV, Webb, PA, Murphy, FA. Isolation and Partial Characterisation of a New Virus Causing Acute Haemorrhagic Fever in Zaire. *Lancet* I, 569–71. 1977; Bowen, ETW, Lloyd, G, Harris, WJ, Platt, GS, Baskerville, A, Vella, EE. Viral Haemorrhagic Fever in Southern Sudan and Northern Zaire. *Lancet* I, 571. 1977; Pattyn, S, Van Der Groen, G, Jacob, W, Piot, P, Courteille, G. Isolation of Marburg-like Virus from a Case of Haemorrhagic Fever in Zaire. *Lancet* I, 573. 1977.

6 Emond, RTD, Evans, B, Bowen, ETW, Lloyd, G. A Case of Ebola Virus Infection. *BMJ* 2, 541–4. 1977.

7 Formenty, P, Boesch, C, Wyers, M, Steiner, C, et al. Ebola Virus Outbreak Among Wild Chimpanzees Living in a Rain Forest of Côte d'Ivoire. *JID* 179(Suppl 1): S120–126. 1999.

8 Formenty, P, Hatz, C, Le Guenno, B, Stoll, A, et al. Human Infection Due to Ebolavirus, Subtype Côte d'Ivoire: Clinical and Biological Presentation. *JID* 179(Suppl 1): S48–53. 1999.

9 Le Guenno, B, Formentry, P, Wyers, M, Gounon, P, Walker, F, Boesch, C. Isolation and Partial Characterisation of a New Strain of Ebola Virus. *Lancet* 345: 1271–4. 1995.

10 Towner, JS, Sealy, TK, Khristova, ML, Albarino, CG, et al. Newly Discovered Ebola Virus Associated with Hemorrhagic Fever Outbreak in Uganda. PLOS Pathogens 4, issue 11, e1000212. 2008; MacNeil, A, Farnon, EC, Wamala, J, Okware, S, et al. Proportion of Deaths and Clinical Features in Bundibugyo Ebola Virus Infection, Uganda. *Emerging Infectious Diseases* 16, 1969–72. 2010.

11 Becquart, P, Wauquier, N, Mahlakoiv, T, Nkoghe, D, et al. High Prevalence of Both Humeral and Cellular Immunity to *Zaire ebola virus* Among Rural Populations in Gabon. PLoS ONE 5, e9126. 2010.

12 Gonzales, JP, Nakoune, E, Slenczka, W, Vidal, P, Morvam, JM. Ebola and Marburg Antibody Prevalence in Selected Populations of the Central African Republic. *Microbes Infect* 2, 39–44. 2000.

13 Jahrling, PB, Geisbert, TW, Dalgard, DW, Johnson, ED, et al. Preliminary Report: Isolation of Ebola Virus from Monkeys Imported to USA. *Lancet* 335, 502–5. 1990.

14 Miranda, MEG, White, ME, Dayrit, MM, Hayes, CG, et al. Seroepidemiological Study of Filovirus Related to Ebola in the Philippines. *Lancet* 337; 425–6. 1991.

15 Kobinger, GP, Leung, A, Neufeld, J, Richardson, JS, et al. Replication, Pathogenicity, Shedding, and Transmission of *Zaire ebolavirus* in Pigs. *JID* 204; 200–8. 2011.

16 Misasi, J, Sullivan, NJ. Camouflage and Misdirection: The Full-on Assault of Ebolavirus Disease. *Cell* 159, 477–86. 2014.

17 Wauquier, N, Becquart, P, Padilla, C, Baize, S, Leroy, EM. Human Fatal Zaire Ebola Virus Infection is Associated with an Aberrant Innate Immunity and with Massive Lymphocyte Apoptosis. Plos Neglected Tropical Diseases, 4. E837. 2010.

18 Towner, JS, Amman, BR, Sealy, TK, Reeder Carroll, SA, et al. Isolation of Genetically Diverse Marburg Virus from Egyptian Fruit Bats. Plos Pathog 5:e 1000536. 2009.

19 Amman, BR, Jones, ME, Sealy, TK, Uebelhoer, LS, et al. Oral Shedding of Marburg Virus in Experimentally Infected Egyptian Fruit Bats *Rousettus aegyptiacus* J Wildl. Dis. 51; 113–24. 2015.

CHAPTER 3

1 Heymann, DL. Ebola: Learn from the Past. *Nature* 514; 299–300. 2014.

2 Heymann, DL, Weisfeld, JS, Webb, A, Johnson, KM, Cairns, T, Berquist, H. Ebola Hemorrhagic Fever: Tandala, Zaire, 1977–78. *JID* 142; 372–6. 1980.

3 Nkoghe, D, Formenty, P, Leroy, EM, Nhegue, S, et al. Multiple Ebola Virus Haemorrhagic Fever Outbreaks in Gabon, from October 2001 to April 2002. In Bull. *Soc Pantol Exot* 98(3); 224–9. 2005.

4 Leroy, EM, Rouquet, P, Formenty, P, Souuquiere, S, et al. Multiple Ebola Virus Transmission Events and Rapid Decline of Central African Wildlife. *Science* 303; 387–90. 2004.

5 Leroy, EM, Rouquet, P, Formenty, P, Souuquiere, S, et al. Multiple Ebola Virus Transmission Events and Rapid Decline of Central African Wildlife. *Science* 303; 387–90. 2004.

6 Okware, SI, Omaswa, FG, Zaramba, S, et al. An Outbreak of Ebola in Uganda. *Tropical Medicine and International Health* 7; 1068–75. 2002.

7 www.patientsafetyed.duhs.duke.edu/module_e/swiss_cheese.html

8 Ebola Haemorrhagic Fever in Sudan, 1976. Report of a WHO/international study team. Bulletin of the WHO, 56(2): 247–70. 1978.

9 Khan, AS, Tshioko, FK, Heymann, DL, Le Guenno, B, et al. The Re-emergence of Ebola Hemorrhagic Fever, Democratic Republic of Congo, 1995. *JID* 179(Suppl 1); S76–86. 1999.

10 Muyembe-Tamfum, JJ, Kipasa, M, Kiyungu, C, Colebunders, R. Ebola Outbreak in Kikwit, Democratic Republic of Congo: Discovery and Control Measures. *JID* 178(Suppl 1): S259–262. 1999.

11 Honigsbaum, M. Jean-Jacques Muyembe-Tamfum: Africa's Veteran Ebola Hunter. *Lancet* 385; 2455. 2015.

12 Honigsbaum, M. Jean-Jacques Muyembe-Tamfum: Africa's Veteran Ebola Hunter. *Lancet* 385; 2455. 2015.

13 Kibadi, K, Mupapa, K, Kuvula, K, Massamba, M, et al. Late Ophthalmological Manifestations in Survivors of the 1995 Ebola Virus Epidemic in Kikwit, Democratic Republic of the Congo. *JID* 178(Suppl 1): S13–14. 1999.

14 Rowe, AK, Bertolli, J, Khan, AS, Mukunu, R, et al. Clinical, Virologic, and Immunologic Follow-up of Convalescent Ebola Hemorrhagic Fever Patients and their Household Contacts, Kikwit, Democratic Republic of the Congo. *JID* 179(Suppl 1): S28–35. 1999.

15 Heymann, DL, Barakamfitiye, D, Szczeniowski, M, Muyembe-Tamfum, J-J, et al. Ebola Hemorrhagic Fever: Lessons from Kikwit, Democratic Republic of the Congo. *JID* 178(Suppl 1): S283–286. 1999.

16 Muyembe-Tamfum, JJ, Kipasa, M, Kiyungu, C, Colebunders, R. Ebola Outbreak in Kikwit, Democratic Republic of Congo: Discovery and Control Measures. *JID* 178(Suppl 1): S259–262. 1999.

17 Heymann, DL, Barakamfitiye, D, Szczeniowski, M, Muyembe-Tamfum, J-J, et al. Ebola Hemorrhagic Fever: Lessons from Kikwit, Democratic Republic of the Congo. *JID* 178(Suppl 1): S283–286. 1999.

18 Leroy, EM, Kumulungui, B, Pourrut, X, Rouquet, P, et al. Fruit Bats as Reservoirs of Ebola Virus. *Nature* 438, 575–6. 2005.

19 Heyman, DTS, Emmerich, P, yu M, Wang, L-F, Suu-Ire, R, et al. Long-term Survival of an Urban Fruit Bat Seropositive for Ebola and Lagos Bat Viruses. *Plos one*, 5: e11978. 2010.

20 Haymann, DTS, Yu M, Crameri, G, Wang, L-F, et al. Ebola Virus Antibodies in Fruit Bats, Ghana, West Africa. *Emerging Infectious Diseases* 18; 1207–9. 2012.

21 Leroy, EM, Kumulungui, B, Pourrut, X, Rouquet, P, et al. Fruit Bats as Reservoirs of Ebola Virus. *Nature* 438, 575–6. 2005.

22 Amman, BR, Jones, ME, Sealy, TK, Uebelhoer, LS, et al. Oral Shedding of Marburg Virus in Experimentally Infected Egyptian Fruit Bats *Rousettus aegyptiacus* J Wildl. Dis. 51; 113–24. 2015.

23 Pigott, DM, Golding, N, Mylne, A, Huang, Z, et al. Mapping the Zoonotic Niche of Ebola Virus Disease in Africa. *eLife* e04395. 2014.

CHAPTER 4

1 Davies, BC, Bowley, D, Roper K. Response to the Ebola Crisis in Sierra Leone. *Nursing Standard* 29: 37–41. 2015.
2 The Bible. Matthew 24:7–13.
3 Davies, BC, Bowley, D, Roper K. Response to the Ebola Crisis in Sierra Leone. *Nursing Standard* 29: 37–41. 2015.
4 www.bbc.co.uk/news/world-africa-29256443.
5 Hayden, EC. Ebola Doctor. *Nature* 516; 314. September 2014.
6 Birrell, I. The Power of Public Service. *The Independent* 13; December 29, 2014.
7 www.nytimes.com/2014/10/30/opinion/charles-blow-the-ebola-hysteria.html?_r=0. Accessed October 2015.

CHAPTER 5

1 WHO Ebola Response Team. Ebola Virus Disease in West Africa—The First 9 Months of the Epidemic and Forward Projections. *N Engl J Med* 371; 1481–95. 2014.
2 WHO Ebola Response Roadmap. www.who.int/csr/resources/publications/ebola/response-roadmap/en/. Accessed August 2014.
3 Faye, O, Boëlle, P-Y, Heleze, E, Faye, O, et al. Chains of Transmission and Control of Ebola Virus Disease in Conakry, Guinea, in 2014: An Observational Study. *Lancet Infect Dis* 15; 320–6. 2015.
4 Whitty, CJM, Farrar, J, Ferguson, N, Edmunds, WJ, et al. Tough Choices to Reduce Ebola Transmission. *Nature* 515; 192–4. 2014.
5 www.telegraph.co.uk/news/worldnews/ebola/11417690/Meet-the-British-army-officer-helping-to-spearhead-Sierra-Leones-(web page no longer available). Accessed August 2014.
6 Whitty, CJM, Farrar, J, Ferguson, N, Edmunds, WJ, et al. Tough Choices to Reduce Ebola Transmission. *Nature* 515; 192–4. 2014.
7 Kucharski, AJ, Camacho, A, Checchi, F, Waldman, R, et al. Evaluation of the Benefits and Risks of Introducing Community Care Centres, Sierra Leone. *Emerging Infectious Diseases* 21; 393–9. 2015.
8 Kucharski, AJ, Camacho, A, Checchi, F, Waldman, R, et al. Evaluation of the Benefits and Risks of Introducing Community Care Centres, Sierra Leone. *Emerging Infectious Diseases* 21; 393–9. 2015.
9 Manson, K, Knight, J. *Sierra Leone* P 92. Bradt Travel Guide Ltd, UK. ISBN-13 978 1 84162 412 9.
10 www.apps.who.int/ebola/en/ebola-situation-report/situation-reports/ebola-situation-report-28-january-2015.

11 www.msf.org.uk/sites/uk/files/26863_msf_dispatches_autumn_ magazine_uk_web.pdf. Accessed 2015.

CHAPTER 6

1 Ebola: We Must Finish the Job. MSF Operational Update. July 17, 2015.
2 Liu, J. Finish the Fight Against Ebola. *Nature* 524; 27–9. 2015.
3 www.who.int/csr/resources/publications/ebola/ebola-response-phase3/en/. Accessed September 2015.
4 Blackley, DJ, Lindblade, KA, Kateh, F, Broyles, LN, et al. Rapid Intervention to Reduce Transmission in a Remote Village—Gbarpolu County, Liberia, 2014. *MMWR* 64/N07; 175–8. 2015; Nyenswah, T, Blackley, DJ, Freeman, T, Lindblade, KA, et al. Community Quarantine to Interrupt Ebola Virus Transmission—Mawah Village, Bong County, Liberia, August–October, 2014. *MMWR* 64/N07; 179–82. 2015.
5 www.who.int/csr/resources/publications/ebola/ebola-response-phase3/en/. Accessed September 2015.
6 www.apps.who.int/ebola/current-situation/ebola-situation-report-8-july-2015; www.apps.who.int/ebola/current-situation/ebola-situation-report-15-july-2015.
7 Bausch, DG, Towner, JS, Dowell, SF, et al. Assessment of the Risk of Ebola Virus Transmission from Bodily Fluids and Fomites. J Infect Dis. 196; S142–147. 2007; Rodriguez, LL, De Roo, A, Guimand Y, et al. Persistence and Genetic Stability of Ebola Virus During the Outbreak in Kikwit, Democratic Republic of Congo,1995. *JID* 179(Suppl 1): S170–176. 1999.
8 Rodriguez, LL, De Roo, A, Guimand Y et al. Persistence and genetic stability of Ebola virus during the outbreak in Kikwit, Democratic Republic of Congo,1995. *JID* 179(Suppl 1): S170–176. 1999.
9 Deen, GF, Knust, B, Sesay, FR, et al. Ebola RNA Persistence in Semen of Ebola Virus Disease Survivors—Preliminary Report. *N Engl J Med* DOI: 10.1056/NEJMoa1511410.
10 Christie, A, Davies-Wayne, GJ, Cordier-Lasalle, T, et al. Possible Sexual Transmission of Ebola Virus—Liberia, 2015. *MMWR* 64; 479–81. 2015.
11 Mate, SE, Kugelman, JR, Nyenswah, TG, et al. Molecular Evidence of Sexual Transmission of Ebola Virus. *N Engl J Med* DOI: 10.1056/NEJMoa1509773. Accessed 2015.

12 www.who.int/reproductivehealth/topics/rtis/ebola-virus-semen /en/. Accessed May 2015.

13 Clark, DV, Kibuuka, H, Millard, M, et al. Long-term Sequelae After Ebola Virus Disease in Bundibuagyo, Uganda: A Retrospective Study. *Lancet Infect Dis* 15; 905–12. 2015.

14 Sukel, K. I Would Have Been Dead in a Week. *New Scientist* Opinion Interview, 26. 6 June 2015.

15 Sukel, K. I Would Have Been Dead in a Week. *New Scientist* Opinion Interview, 26. 6 June 2015.

16 Varkey, JB, Shantha, JG, Crozier, I, et al. Persistence of Ebola Virus in Ocular Fluid During Convalescence. *New Engl J Med* 372; 2423–7. 2015.

17 Sukel, K. I Would Have Been Dead in a Week. *New Scientist* Opinion Interview, 29. 6 June 2015.

18 Ebola Workers 'Always at Risk'. *Sunday Times* October 18, 2015.

19 Jacobs, M, Rodger, A, Bell, D, Bhagani, S, et al. A Case of Late Ebola Virus Relapse Causing Meningoencephalitis. *Lancet*, 338, 498–503. 2016.

20 www.theguardian.com/world/2015/nov/12/ebola-nurse-pauline-cafferkey-glasgow.

21 Reardon, S. Ebola's Mental-health Wounds Linger in Africa. *Nature* 519: 13–14. 2015.

22 Evans, DK and Popova, A. West Africa Ebola Crisis and Orphans. *Lancet* 385; 945–6. 2015.

23 Liberia: Counting the Cost of the Ebola Outbreak. www.msf.org/ article/liberia-counting-cost-ebola-outbreak. Accessed May 2015.

24 Hayden, EC. Ebola's Lasting Legacy. *Nature* 519; 24–6. 2015.

25 Baggi, FM, Taybi, A, Kurth, A, et al. Management of Pregnant Women Infected with Ebola Virus in a Treatment Centre in Guinea. www. eurosurveillance.org/ViewArticle.aspx?ArticleId=20983. Accessed December 2014.

26 Walker, PGT, White, MT, Griffin, JT, et al. Malaria Morbidity and Mortality in Ebola-affected Countries Caused by Decreased Health-care Capacity, and the Potential Effect of Mitigation Strategies: A Modelling Analysis. *Lancet* 15: 825–32. 2015.

27 Plucinski, MM, Guilavogui, T, Sidikiba, S, et al. Effect of Ebola-virus-disease Epidemic on Malaria Case Management in Guinea, 2014: A Cross-sectional Survey of Health Facilities. *Lancet Infect Dis* 15: 1017–23. 2015.

28 Walker, PGT, White, MT, Griffin, JT, et al. Malaria Morbidity and Mortality in Ebola-affected Countries Caused by Decreased Health-care Capacity, and the Potential Effect of Mitigation Strategies: A Modelling Analysis. *Lancet* 15: 825–32. 2015.

29 www.who.int/malaria/publications/atoz/malaria-control-ebola-affected-countries/en/.

30 Walker, PGT, White, MT, Griffin, JT, et al. Malaria Morbidity and Mortality in Ebola-affected Countries Caused by Decreased Health-care Capacity, and the Potential Effect of Mitigation Strategies: A Modelling Analysis. *Lancet* 15: 825–32. 2015.

31 Pringle, J, Kuehne, A, Janssens, M, Pratt, O, et al. Mass Drug Administration of Antimalarials in the Ebola Epidemic in Sierra Leone and Liberia. www.msf.org.uk/sites/uk/files/2_56_pringle_ebola_ocba_sv_final.pdf. Accessed March 2015.

CHAPTER 7

1 Baize, S, Pannetier, D, Oestereich, L, Rieger, T, et al. Emergence of Zaire Ebola Virus Disease in Guinea. *N Engl J Med* 371; 1418–25. 2014.

2 Saéz, AM, Weiss, S, Nowak, K, Lapeyre, V, et al. Investigating the Zoonotic Origin of the West African Ebola Epidemic. *EMBO molecular medicine* 7: 17–23. 2015.

3 Pourrut, X, Souris, M, Towner, JS, Rollin, P, et al. Large Serological Survey Showing Cocirculation of Ebola and Marburg Viruses in Gabonese Bat Populations, and a High Seroprevalence of Both Viruses in *Rousettus aegyptiacus*. *BMC Infectious Diseases* 9; 159–69. 2009.

4 WHO Ebola Response Team. Ebola Virus Disease in West Africa—The First 9 Months of the Epidemic and Forward Projections. *N Engl J Med* 371; 1481–95. 2014.

5 Carroll, MW, Matthews, DA, Hiscox, JA, Pollakis, G, et al. Temporal and Spatial Analysis of the 2014–2015 Ebola Virus Outbreak in West Africa. *Nature* 524; 97–101. 2015.

6 Gire, SK, Goba, A, Andersen, KG, Sealfon, RSG, et al. Genomic Surveillance Elucidates Ebola Virus Origin and Transmission During the 2014 Outbreak. *Science* 345; 1369–72. 2014; Baize, S, Pannetier, D, Oestereich, L, Rieger, T, et al. Emergence of Zaire Ebola Virus Disease in Guinea. *N Engl J Med* 371; 1418–25. 2014.

7 Gire SK, Goba A, Andersen KG, Sealfon RSG et al. Genomic surveillance elucidates Ebola virus Origin and Transmission During the

2014 Outbreak. *Science* 345; 1369–72; Simon-Loriere, E, Faye, O, Koivogui, L, et al. Distinct Lineages of Ebola Virus in Guinea During The 2014 West African Epidemic. *Nature* 524; 102–4. 2015; Tong, Y-G, Shi, W-F, Liu, D, Qian, J, et al. Genetic Diversity and Evolutionary Dynamics of Ebola Virus in Sierra Leone. *Nature* 524; 93–6. 2015.

8 Gire, SK, Goba, A, Andersen, KG, Sealfon, RSG, et al. Genomic Surveillance Elucidates Ebola Virus Origin and Transmission During the 2014 Outbreak. *Science* 345; 1369–72.

9 Carroll, MW, Matthews, DA, Hiscox, JA, Pollakis, G, et al. Temporal and Spatial Analysis of the 2014–2015 Ebola Virus Outbreak in West Africa. *Nature* 524; 97–101. 2015; Simon-Loriere, E, Faye, O, Koivogui, L, et al. Distinct Lineages of Ebola Virus in Guinea During the 2014 West African Epidemic. *Nature* 524; 102–4. 2015; Tong, Y-G, Shi, W-F, Liu, D, Qian, J, et al. Genetic Diversity and Evolutionary Dynamics of Ebola Virus in Sierra Leone. *Nature* 524; 93–6. 2015; Ladner, JT, Wiley, MR, Kate, S, et al. Evolution and Spread of Ebola Virus in Liberia 2014–2015. *Cell Host Microbe* 18; 659–69. 2015; Park, DJ, Dudas, G, Wohl, S, Rambaut, A, Garry, RF, Sabeti, PC, et al. Ebola Virus Epidemiology, Transmission, and Ebola Evolution During Seven Months in Sierra Leone. *Cell* 161; 1516–26. 2015.

10 Sack, K, Fink, S, Belluck, P, Nossiter, A. How Ebola Roared Back. www.nytimes.com/2014/12/30/health/how-ebola-roared-back. html?_r=0. Accessed December 2014.

11 Moon, S, Sridhar, D, Pate, MA, et al. Will Ebola Change the Game? Ten Essential Reforms Before the Next Pandemic. The Report of the Harvard-LSHTM Independent Panel on the Global Response to Ebola. *Lancet* 386; 2204–3321. 2015.

CHAPTER 8

1 Sterk E. Filovirus Haemorrhagic Fever Guideline. Médècins Sans Frontières. www.medbox.org/filovirus-haemorrhagic-fever-guide-line. Accessed 2008.

2 Bah, EI, Lamah, M-C, Fletcher, T, et al. Clinical Presentation of Patients with Ebola Virus Disease in Conakry, Guinea. *N Engl J Med* 372; 40–7. 2015.

3 Lyon, GM, Mehta, AK, Varkey, JB, et al. Clinical Care of Two Patients with Ebola Virus Disease in the United States. *N Engl J Med* 371; 2402–8. 2014.

4 Cohen, J, Enserink, M. Special Report: Ebola's Thin Harvest. www.scim.ag/ThinHarvest; Cohen, J, Enseribk, M. As Ebola Epidemic Draws to a Close, a Thin Scientific Harvest. *Science* 351; 12–13. 2016.

5 Van Griensven, J, Edwards, T, de Lamballerie, X, et al. Evaluation of Convalescent Plasma for Ebola Virus Disease in Guinea. *N Engl J Med* 374; 33–42. 2016.

6 Zhang, YF, Li, DP, Jin, X, Huang, Z. Fighting Ebola with ZMapp: Spotlight on Plant-made Antibody. *Sci China Life Sci* 57; 987–8. 2014.

7 Qui, X, Wong, G, Audet, J, et al. Reversion of Advanced Ebola Virus Disease in Nonhuman Primates with ZMapp. *Nature* 514; 47–53. 2014.

8 www.who.int/mediacentre/news/statements/2014/ebola-ethical-review-summary/en/.

9 Lanini, S, Zumla, A, Ioannidis, JPA, et al. Are Adaptive Randomised Trials or Non-randomised Studies the Best Way to Address the Ebola Outbreak in West Africa. *Lancet Infect Dis* 15; 738–45. 2015.

10 Farrar, J, Heymann, D, Piot, P. Experimental Medicine in a Time of Ebola. *The Wall Street Journal.* August 6, 2014.

11 Cohen, J, Enserink, M. Special Report: Ebola's Thin Harvest. www.scim.ag/ThinHarvest; Cohen, J, Enserink, M. As Ebola Epidemic Draws to a Close, a Thin Scientific Harvest. *Science* 351; 12–13. 2016.

12 Davey, RT. PREVAIL II: A Randomised Controlled Trial of ZMapp in Acute Ebola Virus Infection. Conference on Retroviruses and Opportunistic Infections. Abstract 77LB. February 2016.

13 Oestereich, L, Lüdtke, A, Wurr, S, Rieger, T, Muñoz-Fontela, C, Günter, S. Successful Treatment of Advanced Ebola Virus Infection with T-705 (favipiravir) in a Small Animal Model. *Antiviral Research* 105; 17–21. 2014.

14 www.msf.org/article/preliminary-results-jiki-clinical-trial-test-efficacy-favipiravir-reducing-mortality; Cohen, J, Enserink, M. Special Report: Ebola's Thin Harvest. www.summary/en/:// scim.ag/ ThinHarvest. Accessed December 2015; Sissoko, D, Folfesson, E, Abdoul, M, et al. Favipiravir in Patients with Ebola Virus Disease: Early Results of the JIKI Trial in Guinea. Conference on Retroviruses and Opportunistic Infections. Abstract 103-ALB. February 2015.

15 Dunning, J, Sahr, F, Rojek, A, et al. Experimental Treatment of Ebola Virus Disease with TKM-130803: A Single-arm Phase 2 Trial. PLOS medicine DOI 10. 1371/journal.pmed.1001997. 2016.

16 Gignoux, E, Azman, AS, de Smet, M, et al. Effect of Artesunate-Amodiaquine on Mortality to Ebola Virus Disease. *N Engl J Med* 374; 23–32. 2016.

17 Stanley, DA, Honko, AN, Asiedu, C, et al. Chimpanzee Adenovirus Vaccine Generated Acute and Durable Protective Immunity Against Ebolavirus Challenge. *Nature med* 20; 1126–31. 2014; Geisbert, TW, Feldmann, H. Recombinant Vesicular Stomatitis Virus-Based Vaccines Against Ebola and Marburg Virus Infections. *J Infect Dis* 204; S1075-S1081. 2011.

18 Ledgerwood, JE, DeZure, AD, Stanley, DA, et al. Chimpanzee Adenovirus Vector Ebola Vaccine—Preliminary Report. November 26, 2014 DOI: 10.1056/NEJMoa1410863.

19 Agnandji, ST, Huttner, A, Zinser, ME, et al. Phase 1 Trials of rVSV Ebola Vaccine in Africa and Europe—Preliminary Report. April 1, 2015 DOI: 10.1056/NEJMoa1502924.

20 www.niaid.nih.gov/news/QA/Pages/EbolaVaxresultsQA.aspx. Accessed February 2015.

21 Meltzer, MI, Atkins, CY, Santibanez, S, et al. Estimating the Future Number of Cases in the Ebola Epidemic—Liberia and Sierra Leone, 2014–2015. *MMWR* 63; 1–14. 2014.

22 www.cdc.gov/vhf/ebola/strive/qa.html. Accessed December 2015.

23 Ebola ça Suffit Ring Vaccination Trial Consortium. The Ring Vaccination Trial: A Novel Cluster Randomised Controlled Trial Design to Evaluate Vaccine Efficacy and Effectiveness During Outbreaks, with Special Reference for Ebola. *BMJ* 351; h3740. 2015.

24 Henao-Restrepo, AM, Longini, IM, Egger, M, et al. Efficacy and Effectiveness of an rVSV-Vectored Vaccine Expressing Ebola Surface Glycoprotein: Interim Results from the Guinea Ring Vaccination Cluster-randomised Trial. *Lancet* 386; 857–66. 2015.

25 Henao-Restrepo, AM, Longini, IM, Egger, M, et al. Efficacy and Effectiveness of an rVSV-Vectored Vaccine Expressing Ebola Surface Glycoprotein: Interim Results from the Guinea Ring Vaccination Cluster-randomised Trial. *Lancet* 386; 857–66. 2015.

26 www.who.int/mediacentre/events/2015/S2.1_Janssen_ZEBOV_vaccine-Revised.pdf. Accessed January 2015.

CHAPTER 9

1 Personal communication. Abigail Kent. UK Government Department for International Development. 2015.

2 Moon, S, Sridhar, D, Pate, MA, et al. Will Ebola Change The Game? Ten Essential Reforms Before the Next Pandemic. The Report of the

Harvard–LSHTM Independent Panel on the Global Response to Ebola. *Lancet* 386; 2204–3321. 2015.

3 Advisory Group on Reform of WHO's Work in Outbreaks and Emergencies. Second Report. January 18, 2016. www.who.int/about/who_reform/emergency-capacities/advisory-group/second-report.pdf?ua=1.

4 Kupferschmidt, K. Crisis Manager with 194 Bosses. *Science* 350; 495. 2015.

5 Moon, S, Sridhar, D, Pate, MA et al. Will Ebola Change the Game? Ten Essential Reforms Before the Next Pandemic. The Report of the Harvard–LSHTM Independent Panel on the Global Response to Ebola. *Lancet* 386; 2204–3321. 2015.

6 Moon, S, Sridhar, D, Pate, MA, et al. Will Ebola Change The Game? Ten Essential Reforms Before the Next Pandemic. The Report of the Harvard–LSHTM Independent Panel on the Global Response to Ebola. *Lancet* 386; 2204–3321. 2015.

7 Broadhurst, MJ, Kelly, JD, Miller, A, et al. ReEBOV Antigen Rapid Test Kit for Point-of-care and Laboratory-based Testing for Ebola Virus Disease: A Field Validation Study. *Lancet* 386; 867–74. 2015.

8 Callaway, E. Ebola Hunters Go After Viral Hideouts. *Nature* 529; 138–9. 2016.

9 Plotkin, SA, Mahmoud, AAF, Farrar, J. Establishing a Global Vaccine-development Fund. *N Engl J Med* 373; 297–300. 2015.

POSTSCRIPT

1 Enserink, M. An Obscure Mosquito-borne Disease Goes Global. *Science* 350; 1012–13. 2015.

2 Gates, B. The Next Epidemic—Lessons from Ebola. New Engl J Med 372; 1381–4. 2015.

INDEX

Tables, figures, and glossary items are indicated by an italic *t*, *f*, and *g* following the page number.

DEADLY COMPANIONS

How microbes shaped our history

Dorothy H. Crawford

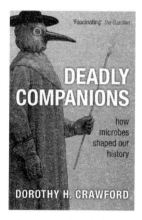

978-0-19-956144-5 | Paperback | £9.99

"Admirably clear and engaging."

BBC History

Ever since we started huddling together in communities, the story of human history has been inextricably entwined with the story of microbes. They have evolved and spread amongst us, shaping our culture through infection, disease, and pandemic. At the same time, our changing human culture has itself influenced the evolutionary path of microbes.

In *Deadly Companions*, Dorothy Crawford examines how the way we live our lives today – with increasing crowding and air travel – puts us once again at risk and asks whether we might ever conquer microbes completely, or whether we need to take a more microbe-centric view of the world. Among the possible answers, one thing becomes clear: that for generations to come, our deadly companions will continue to shape human history.

SPITTING BLOOD

The History of Tuberculosis

Helen Bynum

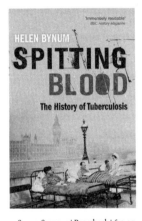

978-0-19-872751-4 | Paperback | £10.99

"Helen Bynum has written a book not only full of diverting asides but also of urgent importance."

Richard Horton, *The Guardian*

Tuberculosis is characterized as a social disease and few have been more inextricably linked with human history. There is evidence from the archaeological record that *Mycobacterium tuberculosis* and its human hosts have been together for a very long time. The very mention of tuberculosis brings to mind romantic images of great literary figures pouring out their souls in creative works as their bodies were being decimated by consumption.

From the medieval period to the modern day, Helen Bynum explores the history and development of tuberculosis throughout the world, touching on the various discoveries that have emerged about the disease over time, and examines the place tuberculosis holds in the popular imagination and its role in various forms of the dramatic arts.

THE INVISIBLE ENEMY

A Natural History of Viruses

Dorothy Crawford

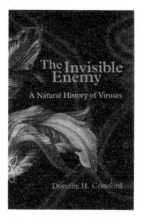

978-0-19-856481-2 | Paperback | £11.99

"The book is lovingly researched and packed with fascinating anecdotes and I found it extremely difficult to put down…No home is complete without this book, if only as a reminder to wash your hands."

Press and Journal

Viruses are disarmingly small and simple. None the less, the smallpox virus killed over 300 million people in the 20th century prior to its eradication in 1980. The AIDS virus, HIV, is now the single most common cause of death in Africa. In recent years, the outbreaks of several lethal viruses such as Ebola and hanta virus have caused great public concern.

In *The Invisible Enemy*, Dorothy Crawford describes all aspects of the natural history of these deadly parasites, explaining how they differ from other microorganisms. She looks at the havoc viruses have caused in the past, where they have come from, and the detective work involved in uncovering them. Finally, she considers whether a new virus could potentially wipe out the human race.